United States Department of Agriculture

Agricultural Research Service

Home and Garden Bulletin Number 72

Nutritive Value of Foods

Susan E. Gebhardt and Robin G. Thomas

U.S. Department of Agriculture, Agricultural Research Service, Nutrient Data Laboratory, Beltsville, Maryland

Abstract

Gebhardt, Susan E., and Robin G. Thomas. 2002. Nutritive Value of Foods. U.S. Department of Agriculture, Agricultural Research Service, Home and Garden Bulletin 72

This publication gives in tabular form the nutritive values for household measures of commonly used foods. It was first published in 1960; the last revision was published in 1991. In this revision, values for total dietary fiber have been added and phosphorus values have been removed. Values are reported for water; calories; protein; total fat; saturated, monounsaturated, and polyunsaturated fatty acids; cholesterol; carbohydrate; total dietary fiber; calcium; iron; potassium; sodium; vitamin A in IU and RE units; thiamin; riboflavin; niacin; and ascorbic acid (vitamin C). Data are from the U.S. Department of Agriculture Nutrient Database for Standard Reference, Release 13.

Keywords: ascorbic acid, calcium, calories, cholesterol, dietary fiber, fatty acids, foods, iron, niacin, nutrient composition, nutrient data, potassium, protein, riboflavin, salt, sodium, total fat, vitamin A

Mention of trade names, commercial products, or companies in this publication is solely for the purpose of providing specific information and does not imply recommendation or endorsement by the U.S. Department of Agriculture over others not mentioned.

Revised October 2002

The U.S. Department of Agriculture (USDA) prohibits discrimination in all its programs and activities on the basis of race, color, national origin, sex, religion, age, disability, political beliefs, sexual orientation, or marital or family status. (Not all prohibited bases apply to all programs.) Persons with disabilities who require alternative means for communication of program information (Braille, large print, audiotape, etc.) should contact USDA's TARGET Center at (202) 720-2600 (voice and TDD).

To file a complaint of discrimination, write USDA, Office of Civil Rights, Room 326-W, Whitten Building, 1400 Independence Avenue, SW, Washington, D.C. 20250-9410 or call (202) 720-5964 (voice and TDD). USDA is an equal opportunity provider and employer

---

For sale by the Superintendent of Documents, U.S. Government Printing Office
Internet: bookstore.gpo.gov Phone: toll free (866) 512-1800; DC area (202) 512-1800
Fax: (202) 512-2250 Mail: Stop SSOP, Washington, DC 20402-0001

ISBN 0-16-051197-6

Contents

Acknowledgments	iv
Abbreviations	v
Introduction	1
Further information	1
Literature cited	2

Tables

1	Equivalents by volume and weight	3
2	Tips for estimating amount of food consume	4
3	Yield of cooked meat per pound of raw meat as purchased	5
4	Recommended daily dietary intakes	6
5	Food sources of additional nutrients	8
6	Daily values	9
7	Amount of total fat that provides 30 percent of calories and saturated fat that provides 10 percent	10
8	Caffeine values	11
9	Nutritive value of the edible part of food	12
	Beverages	14
	Dairy products	16
	Eggs	22
	Fats and oils	22
	Fish and shellfish	26
	Fruits and fruit juices	28
	Grain products	36
	Legumes, nuts, and seeds	52
	Meat and meat products	56
	Mixed dishes and fast foods	60
	Poultry and poultry products	66
	Soups, sauces, and gravies	68
	Sugars and sweets	70
	Vegetables and vegetable products	76
	Miscellaneous items	86
Index for table 9		90

Acknowledgments

The following people deserve special thanks for their roles in this project:

Joanne M. Holden, research leader, Nutrient Data Laboratory

Food specialists of the Nutrient Data Laboratory, all of whom contributed data for the various food groups: Rena Cutrufelli, Vincent De Jesus, Jacob Exler, David Haytowitz, Gwen Holcomb, Juliette Howe, Linda Lemar, Pamela Pehrsson, and Bethany Showell

Dr. Mark Kantor, associate professor and extension specialist, University of Maryland, College Park; Lisa Lachenmayr, extension educator, Maryland Cooperative Extension—Prince George's County; and Kristin Marcoe, nutritionist, USDA Center for Nutrition Policy and Promotion, each of whom reviewed the manuscript and provided helpful comments.

Abbreviations

dia	diameter
fl oz	fluid ounce
g	gram
kcal	kilocalorie (commonly known as calories)
IU	International Units
lb	pound
μg	microgram
mg	milligram
ml	milliliter
NA	not available
oz	ounce
pkg	package
RE	retinol equivalent
sq	square
tbsp	tablespoon
Tr	trace
tsp	teaspoon

Nutritive Value of Foods

by Susan E. Gebhardt and Robin G. Thomas, U.S. Department of Agriculture,
Agricultural Research Service, Nutrient Data Laboratory, Beltsville, Maryland

Introduction

An 8-oz glass of milk, a 3-oz slice of cooked meat, an apple, a slice of bread. What food values does each contain? How much cooked meat will a pound of raw meat yield? How much protein should a healthy 14-year-old boy get each day?

Consumers want ready answers to questions like these so they can plan nutritious diets for themselves and their families. Also, nutritionists, dietitians, and other health professionals use this type of information in their daily work.

In response, the U.S. Department of Agriculture published the first edition of this bulletin in 1960. USDA nutrition researchers have revised it many times since to reflect our expanded knowledge, to add or subtract specific values, and to update the ever-growing list of available, commonly used foods.

Further Information

The USDA Nutrient Database for Standard Reference is a more technical compilation of nutrient information, with data for a much more extensive list of foods and nutrients than this publication provides. It is revised regularly and published on the USDA Nutrient Data Laboratory (NDL) web site, <www.nal.usda.gov/fnic/foodcomp>. It replaces USDA's Agriculture Handbook 8, "Composition of Foods...Raw, Processed, Prepared," commonly referred to as "Handbook 8," and its revised sections, which are out of print. Special-interest tables—such as Isoflavone Content of Foods—are also published on the NDL web site.

The USDA Nutrient Database for Standard Reference and special-interest tables produced by NDL are also available on CD-ROM from the U.S. Government Printing Office (GPO). See the back of the title page for contact information.

Other nutrition publications that may be useful include "Nutrition and Your Health: Dietary Guidelines for Americans," USDA Home and Garden Bulletin 232; "Making Healthy Food Choices," USDA Home and Garden Bulletin 250; and "Check It Out: The Food Label, the Pyramid, and You," USDA Home and Garden Bulletin 266. These publications may also be purchased from GPO. See the back of the title page for contact information.

The Dietary Guidelines for Americans and the Food Guide Pyramid can be found on USDA's Center for Nutrition Policy and Promotion web site, <http://www.usda.gov/cnpp>, or write to them at 3101 Park Center Dr., Room 1064, Alexandria, VA 22302-1594. Food label and other nutrition information can be found on the Food and Drug Administration's Center for Food Safety and Applied Nutrition web site, <http://vm.cfsan.fda.gov/label.html>, or write to them at 200 C Street, SW, Washington, DC 20204.

Full texts of the Recommended Dietary Allowances and each volume of Dietary Reference Intakes are available from the National Academy Press, at www.nap.edu or 888-624-8373 (toll free).

For more information about food and nutrition, visit the USDA-ARS National Agricultural Library's Food and Nutrition Information Center <http://www.nal.usda.gov/fnic/>, or contact them at 10301 Baltimore Ave., Room 304, Beltsville, MD 20705-2351, Phone: 301-504-5719, Fax: 301-504-6409, TTY: 301-504-6856, e-mail: fnic@nal.usda.gov. Another source of information on the Internet is <www.nutrition.gov>.

Literature Cited

American Institute for Cancer Research. 2001. The New American Plate. On the American Institute for Cancer Research web site <www.aicr.org>, page URL: <http://www.aicr.org/nap2.htm> (February 5, 2002).

Schuster, Ellen, compiler. 1997. Making Sense of Portion Sizes. On the Oregon State University Extension Family & Community Development web site <http://osu.orst.edu/dept/ehe/nutrition.htm>, page URL: <http://osu.orst.edu/dept/ehe/nu_n&f_ms.htm> (February 5, 2002).

Standing Committee on the Scientific Evaluation of Dietary Reference Intakes, Food and Nutrition Board, Institute of Medicine. 1997. Dietary Reference Intakes for Calcium, Phosphorus, Magnesium, Vitamin D, and Fluoride. National Academy Press, Washington, D.C.

_____. 1998. Dietary Reference Intakes for Thiamin, Riboflavin, Niacin, Vitamin B6, Folate, Vitamin B12, Pantothenic Acid, Biotin, and Choline. National Academy Press, Washington, D.C.

_____. 2000. Dietary Reference Intakes for Vitamin C, Vitamin E, Selenium, and Carotenoids. National Academy Press, Washington, D.C.

Subcommittee on the Tenth Edition of the RDAs, Food and Nutrition Board, Commission on Life Sciences, National Research Council. 1989. Recommended Dietary Allowances, 10th ed. National Academy Press, Washington, D.C.

U.S. Department of Agriculture, Agricultural Research Service. 2000. USDA Nutrient Database for Standard Reference, Release 13. The Service, Washington, D.C

U.S. Department of Agriculture and U.S. Department of Health and Human Services. 2000. Nutrition and Your Health: Dietary Guidelines for Americans, 5th ed. USDA and DHHS, Home and Garden Bulletin 232.

U.S. Food and Drug Administration. 1999. Food Labeling. Code of Federal Regulations, Title 21, part 101. [Available on the U.S. Government Printing Office web site <http://www.access.gpo.gov)>, 21CFR101 URL: http://www.access.gpo.gov/nara/cfr/waisidx_99/21cfr101_99.html> (February 5, 2002)].

Table 1. Equivalents by Volume and Weight

This table contains some helpful volume and weight equivalents. Following is an example that illustrates how you can use the table:

Example. For milk, the nutrient profile covers a 1-cup serving (see page 20, table 9). Let's say you use 2 tablespoons of milk in your coffee. In table 1, you see that 1 cup equals 16 tablespoons, so the 2 tablespoons you consume are two-sixteenths or one-eighth of 1 cup. To find out the nutritive value of the amount you actually consume—2 tablespoons—you need to divide the nutrient values listed for milk by 8.

Volume

1 gallon (3.786 liters; 3,786 ml)	4 quarts
1 quart (0.946 liter; 946 ml)	4 cups or 2 pints
1 cup (237 ml)	8 fluid ounces, ½ pint, or 16 tablespoons
2 tablespoons (30 ml)	1 fluid ounce
1 tablespoon (15 ml)	3 teaspoons
1 pint	2 cups

Weight

1 pound (16 ounces)	453.6 grams
1 ounce	28.35 grams
3½ ounces	100 grams

Table 2. Tips for Estimating Amount of Food Consumed

This table lists some handy tips to help you estimate the amount of food you eat when you cannot measure or weigh it.

Breads and grains

½ cup cooked cereal, pasta, rice	volume of cupcake wrapper or half a baseball
4-oz bagel (large)	diameter of a compact disc (CD)
medium piece of cornbread	medium bar of soap

Fruits and vegetables

medium apple, orange, peach	tennis ball
¼ cup dried fruit	golf ball or scant handful for average adult
½ cup fruit or vegetable	half a baseball
1 cup broccoli	light bulb
medium potato	computer mouse
1 cup raw leafy greens	baseball or fist of average adult
½ cup	6 asparagus spears, 7 or 8 baby carrots or carrot sticks, or a medium ear of corn

Meat, fish, and poultry, cooked

1 oz	about 3 tbsp meat or poultry
2 oz	small chicken drumstick or thigh
3 oz	average deck of cards, palm of average adult's hand, half of a whole, small chicken breast, medium pork chop

Cheese

1 oz hard cheese	average person's thumb, 2 dominoes, 4 dice

Other

2 tbsp peanut butter	Ping-Pong ball
⅓ cup nuts	level handful for average adult
½ cup	half a baseball or base of computer mouse
1 cup	tennis ball or fist of average adult

Note: The serving size indicated in the Food Guide Pyramid and on food labels is a standardized unit of measure and may not represent the portion of food a person actually eats on one occasion.

Sources: Schuster (1997), American Institute of Cancer Research (2001).

Table 3. Yield of Cooked Meat per Pound of Raw Meat as Purchased

From the time it is purchased to the time it is eaten, meat undergoes certain losses. These include evaporation of moisture and loss of fat in the drippings during cooking and removal of parts such as bone, gristle, and fat before or after cooking.

This table shows, for several retail cuts, the yield of cooked meat from 1 pound of raw meat. Yield is given as ounces of:

Cooked meat with bone and fat
Cooked lean and fat
Cooked lean only

Among the factors influencing meat yield is the proportion of fat and lean. Many cuts have an outside layer of fat extending all or part way around. The thickness of this fat layer varies depending on the cutting and trimming practices in the market. The information on yield in table 3 and on nutritive value in table 9 applies to retail cuts trimmed according to typical market practices. Deposits of fat within a cut may be extensive. They are not usually affected by retail trimming but may be discarded after cooking.

Table 3. Yield of Cooked Meat per Pound of Raw Meat as Purchased

Retail cut and method of cooking	Parts weighed	Yield after cooking, less drippings Weight (oz)
Chops or steaks for broiling or frying		
With bone and relatively large amount fat, such as pork or lamb chops; beef rib; sirloin, or porterhouse steaks	Lean, bone, and fat Lean and fat Lean only	10-12 7-10 5-7
Without bone and with very little fat, such as round of beef or veal steaks	Lean and fat Lean only	12-13 9-12
Ground meat for broiling or frying, such as beef, lamb, or pork patties	Patties	9-13
Roast for oven cooking (no liquid added)		
With bone and relatively large amount of fat, such as beef rib, loin, chuck; lamb shoulder, leg; pork, fresh or cured	Lean, bone, and fat Lean and fat Lean only	10-12 8-10 6-9
Without bone	Lean and fat Lean only	10-12 7-10
Cuts for pot roasting, simmering, braising, stewing		
With bone and relatively large amount of fat, such as beef chuck, pork shoulder	Lean, bone, and fat Lean and fat Lean only	10-11 8-9 6-8
Without bone and with relatively small amount of fat, such as trimmed beef, veal	Lean with adhering fat	9-11

Table 4. Recommended Daily Dietary Intakes

Table 4 shows recommended daily levels of calories and several nutrients essential for maintenance of good nutrition in healthy, normally active persons. The Recommended Dietary Allowances (RDAs) are currently being revised by the National Academy of Sciences. The new recommendations are called Dietary Reference Intakes (DRIs) and include two sets of values that serve as goals for nutrient intake—RDAs and Adequate Intakes (AIs). The right side of table 4 presents the DRIs published in 1997-2000, with AIs indicated by a dagger (†). The left side of the table includes the 1989 RDAs. More detailed information about DRIs may be obtained from the table's sources (see note at end of table). Table 4 includes only the nutrients contained in table 9.

Table 4. Recommended Daily Dietary Intakes

1989 Recommended Dietary Allowances (RDA)						2000 Dietary Reference Intakes (DRI)					
Life-Stage Group	Energy* (kcal)	Protein (g)	Vitamin A (µg RE)	Iron (mg)		Life-Stage Group	Calcium† (mg)	Thiamin (mg)	Riboflavin (mg)	Niacin‡ (mg)	Vitamin C (mg)
Infants (mo)						**Infants** (mo)					
0-6	650	13	375	6		0-6	210	0.2†	0.3†	2†	40†
7-12	850	14	375	10		7-12	270	0.3†	0.4†	4†	50†
Children (yr)						**Children** (yr)					
1-3	1300	16	400	10		1-3	500	0.5	0.5	6	15
4-6	1800	24	500	10		4-8	800	0.6	0.6	8	25
7-10	2000	28	700	10							
Males (yr)						**Males** (yr)					
11-14	2500	45	1000	12		9-13	1300	0.9	0.9	12	45
15-18	3000	59	1000	12		14-18	1300	1.2	1.3	16	75
19-24	2900	58	1000	10		19-30	1000	1.2	1.3	16	90
25-50	2900	63	1000	10		31-50	1000	1.2	1.3	16	90
51+	2300	63	1000	10		51-70	1200	1.2	1.3	16	90
						>70	1200	1.2	1.3	16	90
Females (yr)						**Females** (yr)					
11-14	2200	46	800	15		9-13	1300	0.9	0.9	12	45
15-18	2200	44	800	15		14-18	1300	1.0	1.0	14	65
19-24	2200	46	800	15		19-30	1000	1.1	1.1	14	75
25-50	2200	50	800	15		31-50	1000	1.1	1.1	14	75
51+	1900	50	800	10		51-70	1200	1.1	1.1	14	75
						>70	1200	1.1	1.1	14	75
Pregnancy	+300	60	800	30		**Pregnancy**					
						≤18 yr	1300	1.4	1.4	18	80
						19-50 yr	1000	1.4	1.4	18	85
Lactation						**Lactation**					
1st 6 mo	+500	65	1300	15		≤18 yr	1300	1.4	1.6	17	115
2nd 6 mo	+500	62	1200	15		19-50 yr	1000	1.4	1.6	17	120

* Energy needs shown are based on average size and light-to-moderate activity levels. Individual needs may vary because of sedentary or more physically active lifestyle and/or smaller or larger body size.
† Values represent Adequate Intake.
‡ Expressed as niacin equivalents. 1 mg niacin = 60 mg tryptophan; 0-6 months = preformed niacin, not niacin equivalents.

Note: RDAs and DRIs should not be confused with reference values for food labels established by the U.S. Food and Drug Administration, as follows: vitamin A = 5,000 IU; iron = 18 mg; calcium = 1,000 mg; thiamin = 1.5 mg; riboflavin = 1.7 mg; niacin = 20 mg; vitamin C = 60 mg.

Sources: Adapted, with permission, from Subcommittee on the Tenth Edition of the RDAs (1989) and Standing Committee on the Scientific Evaluation of Dietary Reference Intakes (1997, 1998, 2000).

Table 5. Food Sources of Additional Nutrients

Table 5 lists foods that are of special value in supplying six vitamins and four minerals not shown in tables 4 and 9. Foods are considered to be of special value as a nutrient source if the food serving is high in the nutrient compared with other foods.

Vitamins

Vitamin B-6
Bananas
Fish (most)
Liver
Meat
Nuts and seeds
Potatoes and sweetpotatoes
Poultry
Whole-grain and fortified cereals

Vitamin B-12
Eggs
Fish and shellfish
Fortified cereals
Meat
Milk and milk products
Organ meats

Vitamin D
Egg yolk
Fortified cereals
Fortified milk
Liver
High-fat fish

Vitamin E
Margarine
Nuts and seeds
Peanuts and peanut butter
Vegetable oils
Wheat germ
Whole-grain and fortified cereals

Folate
Dark green vegetables
Dry beans, peas, and lentils
Enriched grain products
Fortified cereals
Liver
Orange juice
Wheat germ
Yeast

Vitamin K
Broccoli
Brussels sprouts
Cabbage
Leafy green vegetables
Mayonnaise
Soybean, canola, and olive oils

Minerals

Iodine
Iodized salt
Saltwater fish and shellfish

Magnesium
Cocoa and chocolate
Dark green vegetables (most)
Dry beans, peas, and lentils
Fish
Nuts and seeds
Peanuts and peanut butter
Whole grains

Phosphorus
Dry beans, peas, and lentils
Eggs
Fish
Meat
Milk and milk products
Nuts and seeds
Poultry
Whole grains

Zinc
Dry beans, peas, and lentils
Meat
Poultry
Seeds
Shellfish
Whole-grain and fortified cereals

Table 6. Daily Values

Daily Values have been established by the Food and Drug Administration as references to help consumers use information on food labels to plan a healthy overall diet. The Daily Values provide a reliable guide for most people. It is helpful to know that a 2,000-calorie level is about right for moderately active women, teenage girls, and sedentary men, and 2,500 calories is the target level for many men, teenage boys, and active women. Many older adults, children, and sedentary women need fewer than 2,000 calories a day and may want to select target levels based on 1,600 calories a day. Some active men and teenage boys and very active women may want to select target levels based on 2,800 calories per day. The Daily Values for sodium and cholesterol are the same for everyone, regardless of total calories consumed, so you do not have to make adjustments based on your caloric needs.

Nutrient	Calories	2,000	2,500
Total fat*	Less than	65 g	80 g
Saturated fat†	Less than	20 g	25 g
Cholesterol	Less than	300 mg	300 mg
Sodium	Less than	2,400 mg	2,400 mg
Total carbohydrate		300 g	375 g
Dietary fiber		25 g	30 g
Potassium		3,500 mg	3,500 mg

* Total fat values are based on 30 percent of calories.
† Saturated fat values are based on 10 percent of calories.

Note. Your Daily Values may be higher or lower depending on your calorie needs. The Daily Values are based on expert dietary advice about how much, or how little, of some key nutrients you should eat each day, depending on whether you eat 2,000 or 2,500 calories a day.

Source: U.S. Food and Drug Administration (1999)

Table 7. Amount of Total Fat That Provides 30 Percent of Calories and Saturated Fat That Provides 10 Percent

Several scientific groups suggest that Americans moderate the amount of fat in their diets. Some recommend that fat be limited to amounts that will provide no more than 30 percent of calories. Table 7 lists the amount of fat that provides 30 percent of calories for diets at different total daily calorie levels. For example, a woman wishing to moderate her fat intake to 30 percent of her 2,000-calorie diet is advised to select foods that total no more than 65 grams of fat per day. She can use table 9 to estimate the grams of fat in the foods she eats.

Table 7 also shows the amount of saturated fat that provides 10 percent of calories for diets at several different daily calorie levels. The amounts of saturated fat are given in upper limits because of that type of fat's ability to raise blood cholesterol levels.

Table 7. Amount of Total Fat That Provides 30 Percent of Calories and Saturated Fat That Provides 10 Percent

Total calories per day	Total fat (g) (no more than 30% of total calories)	Saturated fat (g) (no more than 10% of total calories)
1,600	53	18
2,000*	65	20
2,200	73	24
2,500*	80	25
2,800	93	31

* Percent Daily Values on Nutrition Facts Labels are based on a 2,000-calorie diet. Values for 2,000 and 2,500 calories are rounded to the nearest 5 g to be consistent with the label.

Source: U.S. Department of Agriculture and Department of Health and Human Services (2000).

Table 8. Caffeine Values

Caffeine is a compound found mostly in coffee, tea, cola, cocoa, chocolate, and in foods containing these. Table 8 lists the amounts of caffeine found in these beverages and foods.

Food	Serving size	Caffeine (mg)
Beverages		
Chocolate milk, includes malted milk	8 fl oz	5-8
Chocolate shake	16 fl oz	8
Cocoa, prepared from powder		
Regular	6 fl oz	4-6
Sugar-free	6 fl oz	15
Coffee, regular		
Brewed	6 fl oz	103
Prepared from instant	6 fl oz	57
Coffee, decaffeinated		
Brewed	6 fl oz	2
Prepared from instant	6 fl oz	2
Coffee liqueur	1.5 fl oz	14
Cola or pepper-type, with caffeine	12 fl oz	37
Diet cola, with caffeine	12 fl oz	50
Tea, regular		
Brewed	6 fl oz	36
Instant, prepared	8 fl oz	26-36
Tea, chamomile	6 fl oz	0
Tea, decaffeinated, brewed	6 fl oz	2
Chocolate Foods		
Baking chocolate, unsweetened	1 square (1 oz)	58
Brownies	1	1-3
Candies		
Dark chocolate	1.45-oz bar	30
Milk chocolate bar	1.55-oz bar	11
Semisweet chocolate chips	¼ cup	26-28
Chocolate with other ingredients (nuts, crisped rice, etc.)	about 1.5 oz	3-11
Cereal (containing cocoa)	1 oz	1
Cocoa powder, unsweetened	1 tbsp	12
Cookies (chocolate chip, devil's food, chocolate sandwich)	1	1
Chocolate cupcake with chocolate frosting	1	1-2
Frosting	1/12 pkg (2 tbsp)	1-2
Fudge	1 piece (about ¾ oz)	2-3
Ice cream/frozen yogurt	½ cup	2
Pudding		
Prepared from dry mix	½ cup	3
Ready-to-eat	4 oz	6
Syrup		
Thin-type	1 tbsp	3
Fudge-type	1 tbsp	1

Source: U.S. Department of Agriculture, Agricultural Research Service (2000).

Table 9. Nutritive Value of the Edible Part of Food

Table 9 lists the nutritive values of foods commonly consumed in the United States and makes up the bulk of this publication. The data source is USDA Nutrient Database for Standard Reference, Release 13 (U.S. Department of Agriculture, Agricultural Research Service 2000). See Further Information for more about this database. Most differences in values between this table and the Standard Reference are due to rounding.

Foods are grouped under the following headings:
Beverages
Dairy products
Eggs
Fats and oils
Fish and shellfish
Fruits and fruit juices
Grain products
Legumes, nuts, and seeds
Meat and meat products
Mixed dishes and fast foods
Poultry and poultry products
Soups, sauces, and gravies
Sugars and sweets
Vegetables and vegetable products
Miscellaneous items.

Most of the foods listed are in ready-to-eat form. Some are basic products widely used in food preparation, such as flour, oil, and cornmeal. Most snack foods, a separate food group in the Standard Reference, are found under Grain Products.

Measures and weights. The approximate measure given for each food is in cups, ounces, pounds, some other well-known unit, or a piece of a specified size. The measures do not necessarily represent a serving, but the unit given may be used to calculate a variety of serving sizes. For example, nutrient values are given for 1 cup of applesauce. If the serving you consume is ½ cup, divide the values by 2 or multiply by 0.5.

For fluids, the cup measure refers to the standard measuring cup of 8 fluid ounces. The ounce is one-sixteenth of a pound, unless "fluid ounce" is indicated. The weight of a fluid ounce varies according to the food. If the household measure of a food is listed as 1 ounce, the nutrients are based on a weight of 28.35 grams, rounded to 28 grams in the table. All measure weights are actual weights or rounded to the nearest whole number. See table 2, Tips for Estimating Amount of Food Consumed, for help in determining the size of the portion you actually eat or drink.

The table gives the weight in grams for an approximate measure of each food. The weight applies to only the edible portion (part of food normally eaten), such as the banana pulp without the peel. Some poultry descriptions provide weights for the whole part, such as a drumstick, including skin and/or bone. Keep in mind that the nutritive values are only for the edible portions indicated in the description. For example, item 877, roasted chicken drumstick, indicates a weight of 2.9 oz (82 grams) with the bone and skin. But note that the weight of one drumstick, meat only, is listed as 44 grams (about 1½ oz). So the skin and bone equal 38 grams (82 minus 44). Nutrient values are always given for the gram weight listed in the column Weight—in this case, 44 grams.

Food values. Values are listed for water; calories; protein; total fat; saturated, monounsaturated, and polyunsaturated fatty acids; cholesterol; carbohydrate; total dietary fiber; four minerals (calcium, iron, potassium, and sodium); and five vitamins (vitamin A, thiamin, riboflavin, niacin, and ascorbic acid, or vitamin C). Water content is included because the percentage of moisture is helpful for identification and comparison of many food items. For example, to identify whether the cocoa listed is powder or prepared, you could check the water value, which is much less for cocoa powder. Values are in grams or milligrams except for water, calories, and vitamin A.

Food energy is reported as calories. A calorie is the unit of measure for the amount of energy that protein, fat, and carbohydrate furnish the body. Alcohol also contributes to the calorie content of alcoholic beverages. The official unit of measurement for food energy is actually kilocalories (kcal), but the term "calories" is commonly used in its place. In fact, "calories" is used on the food label.

Vitamin A is reported in two different units: International Units (IU) are used on food labels and in the past for expressing vitamin A activity; Retinol Equivalents (RE) are the units released in 1989 by the Food and Nutrition Board for expressing the RDAs for vitamin A.

Values for calories and nutrients shown in table 9 are the amounts in the part of the item that is customarily eaten—corn without cob, meat without bones, and peaches without pits. Nutrient values are averages for products presented here. Values for some nutrients may vary more widely for specific food items. For example, the vitamin A content of beef liver varies widely, but the values listed in table 9 represent an average for that food.

In some cases, as with many vegetables, values for fat may be trace (Tr), yet there will be numerical values listed for some of the fatty acids. The values for fat have been rounded to whole numbers, unless they are between 0 and 0.5; then they are listed as trace. This definition of trace also applies to the other nutrients in table 9 that are rounded to whole numbers.

Other uses of "trace" in table 9 are:

- For nutrients rounded to one decimal place, values falling between 0 and 0.05 are trace.
- For nutrients rounded to two decimal places, values falling between 0 and 0.005 are trace.

Thiamin, riboflavin, niacin, and iron values in enriched white flours, white bread and rolls, cornmeals, pastas, farina, and rice are based on the current enrichment levels established by the Food and Drug Administration. Enrichment levels for riboflavin in rice were not in effect at press time and are not used in table 9. Enriched flour is used in most home-prepared and commercially prepared baked goods.

Niacin values given are for preformed niacin that occurs naturally in foods. The values do not include additional niacin that may be formed in the body from tryptophan, an essential amino acid in the protein of most foods.

Nutrient values for many prepared items were calculated from the ingredients in typical recipes. Examples are biscuits, cornbread, mashed potatoes, white sauce, and many dessert foods. Adjustments were made for nutrient losses during cooking.

Nutrient values for toast and cooked vegetables do not include any added fat, either during preparation or at the table. Cutting or shredding vegetables may destroy part of some vitamins, especially ascorbic acid. Since such losses are variable, no deduction has been made.

Values for cooked dry beans, vegetables, pasta, noodles, rice, cereal, meat, poultry, and fish are without salt added. If hot cereals are prepared with salt, the sodium content ranges from about 324-374 mg for Malt-O-Meal, Cream of Wheat, and rolled oats. The sodium value for corn grits is about 540 mg; sodium for Wheatena is about 238 mg. Sodium values for canned vegetables labeled as "no salt added" are similar to those listed for the cooked vegetables.

The mineral contribution of water was not considered for coffee, tea, soups, sauces, or concentrated fruit juices prepared with water. Sweetened items contain sugar unless identified as artificially sweetened.

Several manufactured items—including some milk products, ready-to-eat breakfast cereals, imitation cream products, fruit drinks, and various mixes—are included in table 9. Such foods may be fortified with one or more nutrients; the label will describe any fortification. Values for these foods may be based on products from several manufacturers, so they may differ from the values provided by any one source. Nutrient values listed on food labels may also differ from those in table 9 because of rounding on labels.

Nutrient values represent meats after they have been cooked and drained of the drippings. For many cuts, two sets of values are shown: meat including lean and fat parts, and lean meat from which the outer fat layer and large fat pads have been removed either before or after cooking.

In the entries for cheeseburger and hamburger in Mixed Dishes and Fast Foods, "condiments" refers to catsup, mustard, salt, and pepper; "vegetables" refers to lettuce, tomato, onion, and pickle; "regular" is a 2-oz patty, and large is a 4-oz patty (precooked weight).

Table 9. Nutritive Value of the Edible Part of Food

Food No.	Food Description	Measure of edible portion	Weight (g)	Water (%)	Calories (kcal)	Protein (g)	Total fat (g)	Fatty acids Saturated (g)	Mono-unsaturated (g)	Poly-unsaturated (g)
	Beverages									
	Alcoholic									
	Beer									
1	Regular	12 fl oz	355	92	146	1	0	0.0	0.0	0.0
2	Light	12 fl oz	354	95	99	1	0	0.0	0.0	0.0
	Gin, rum, vodka, whiskey									
3	80 proof	1.5 fl oz	42	67	97	0	0	0.0	0.0	0.0
4	86 proof	1.5 fl oz	42	64	105	0	0	0.0	0.0	0.0
5	90 proof	1.5 fl oz	42	62	110	0	0	0.0	0.0	0.0
6	Liqueur, coffee, 53 proof	1.5 fl oz	52	31	175	Tr	Tr	0.1	Tr	0.1
	Mixed drinks, prepared from recipe									
7	Daiquiri	2 fl oz	60	70	112	Tr	Tr	Tr	Tr	Tr
8	Pina colada	4.5 fl oz	141	65	262	1	3	1.2	0.2	0.5
	Wine									
	Dessert									
9	Dry	3.5 fl oz	103	80	130	Tr	0	0.0	0.0	0.0
10	Sweet	3.5 fl oz	103	73	158	Tr	0	0.0	0.0	0.0
	Table									
11	Red	3.5 fl oz	103	89	74	Tr	0	0.0	0.0	0.0
12	White	3.5 fl oz	103	90	70	Tr	0	0.0	0.0	0.0
	Carbonated*									
13	Club soda	12 fl oz	355	100	0	0	0	0.0	0.0	0.0
14	Cola type	12 fl oz	370	89	152	0	0	0.0	0.0	0.0
	Diet, sweetened with aspartame									
15	Cola	12 fl oz	355	100	4	Tr	0	0.0	0.0	0.0
16	Other than cola or pepper type	12 fl oz	355	100	0	Tr	0	0.0	0.0	0.0
17	Ginger ale	12 fl oz	366	91	124	0	0	0.0	0.0	0.0
18	Grape	12 fl oz	372	89	160	0	0	0.0	0.0	0.0
19	Lemon lime	12 fl oz	368	90	147	0	0	0.0	0.0	0.0
20	Orange	12 fl oz	372	88	179	0	0	0.0	0.0	0.0
21	Pepper type	12 fl oz	368	89	151	0	Tr	0.3	0.0	0.0
22	Root beer	12 fl oz	370	89	152	0	0	0.0	0.0	0.0
	Chocolate flavored beverage mix									
23	Powder	2-3 heaping tsp	22	1	75	1	1	0.4	0.2	Tr
24	Prepared with milk	1 cup	266	81	226	9	9	5.5	2.6	0.3
	Cocoa									
	Powder containing nonfat dry milk									
25	Powder	3 heaping tsp	28	2	102	3	1	0.7	0.4	Tr
26	Prepared (6 oz water plus 1 oz powder)	1 serving	206	86	103	3	1	0.7	0.4	Tr
	Powder containing nonfat dry milk and aspartame									
27	Powder	½-oz envelope	15	3	48	4	Tr	0.3	0.1	Tr
28	Prepared (6 oz water plus 1 envelope mix)	1 serving	192	92	48	4	Tr	0.3	0.1	Tr
	Coffee									
29	Brewed	6 fl oz	178	99	4	Tr	0	Tr	0.0	Tr
30	Espresso	2 fl oz	60	98	5	Tr	Tr	0.1	0.0	0.1
31	Instant, prepared (1 rounded tsp powder plus 6 fl oz water)	6 fl oz	179	99	4	Tr	0	Tr	0.0	Tr

*Mineral content varies depending on water source.

Choles-terol (mg)	Carbo-hydrate (g)	Total dietary fiber (g)	Calcium (mg)	Iron (mg)	Potas-sium (mg)	Sodium (mg)	Vitamin A (IU)	Vitamin A (RE)	Thiamin (mg)	Ribo-flavin (mg)	Niacin (mg)	Ascor-bic acid (mg)	Food No.
0	13	0.7	18	0.1	89	18	0	0	0.02	0.09	1.6	0	1
0	5	0.0	18	0.1	64	11	0	0	0.03	0.11	1.4	0	2
0	0	0.0	0	Tr	1	Tr	0	0	Tr	Tr	Tr	0	3
0	Tr	0.0	0	Tr	1	Tr	0	0	Tr	Tr	Tr	0	4
0	0	0.0	0	Tr	1	Tr	0	0	Tr	Tr	Tr	0	5
0	24	0.0	1	Tr	16	4	0	0	Tr	0.01	0.1	0	6
0	4	0.0	2	0.1	13	3	2	0	0.01	Tr	Tr	1	7
0	40	0.8	11	0.3	100	8	3	0	0.04	0.02	0.2	7	8
0	4	0.0	8	0.2	95	9	0	0	0.02	0.02	0.2	0	9
0	12	0.0	8	0.2	95	9	0	0	0.02	0.02	0.2	0	10
0	2	0.0	8	0.4	115	5	0	0	0.01	0.03	0.1	0	11
0	1	0.0	9	0.3	82	5	0	0	Tr	0.01	0.1	0	12
0	0	0.0	18	Tr	7	75	0	0	0.00	0.00	0.0	0	13
0	38	0.0	11	0.1	4	15	0	0	0.00	0.00	0.0	0	14
0	Tr	0.0	14	0.1	0	21	0	0	0.02	0.08	0.0	0	15
0	0	0.0	14	0.1	7	21	0	0	0.00	0.00	0.0	0	16
0	32	0.0	11	0.7	4	26	0	0	0.00	0.00	0.0	0	17
0	42	0.0	11	0.3	4	56	0	0	0.00	0.00	0.0	0	18
0	38	0.0	7	0.3	4	40	0	0	0.00	0.00	0.1	0	19
0	46	0.0	19	0.2	7	45	0	0	0.00	0.00	0.0	0	20
0	38	0.0	11	0.1	4	37	0	0	0.00	0.00	0.0	0	21
0	39	0.0	19	0.2	4	48	0	0	0.00	0.00	0.0	0	22
0	20	1.3	8	0.7	128	45	4	Tr	0.01	0.03	0.1	Tr	23
32	31	1.3	301	0.8	497	165	311	77	0.10	0.43	0.3	2	24
1	22	0.3	92	0.3	202	143	4	1	0.03	0.16	0.2	1	25
2	22	2.5	97	0.4	202	148	4	0	0.03	0.16	0.2	Tr	26
1	9	0.4	86	0.7	405	168	5	1	0.04	0.21	0.2	0	27
2	8	0.4	90	0.7	405	173	4	0	0.04	0.21	0.2	0	28
0	1	0.0	4	0.1	96	4	0	0	0.00	0.00	0.4	0	29
0	1	0.0	1	0.1	69	8	0	0	Tr	0.11	3.1	Tr	30
0	1	0.0	5	0.1	64	5	0	0	0.00	Tr	0.5	0	31

Table 9. Nutritive Value of the Edible Part of Food

Food No.	Food Description	Measure of edible portion	Weight (g)	Water (%)	Calories (kcal)	Protein (g)	Total fat (g)	Fatty acids Saturated (g)	Monounsaturated (g)	Polyunsaturated (g)
	Beverages (continued)									
	Fruit drinks, noncarbonated, canned or bottled, with added ascorbic acid									
32	Cranberry juice cocktail	8 fl oz	253	86	144	0	Tr	Tr	Tr	0.1
33	Fruit punch drink	8 fl oz	248	88	117	0	0	Tr	Tr	Tr
34	Grape drink	8 fl oz	250	88	113	0	0	Tr	0.0	Tr
35	Pineapple grapefruit juice drink	8 fl oz	250	88	118	1	Tr	Tr	Tr	0.1
36	Pineapple orange juice drink	8 fl oz	250	87	125	3	0	0.0	0.0	0.0
	Lemonade									
37	Frozen concentrate, prepared	8 fl oz	248	89	99	Tr	0	Tr	Tr	Tr
	Powder, prepared with water									
38	Regular	8 fl oz	266	89	112	0	0	Tr	Tr	Tr
39	Low calorie, sweetened with aspartame	8 fl oz	237	99	5	0	0	0.0	0.0	0.0
	Malted milk, with added nutrients									
	Chocolate									
40	Powder	3 heaping tsp	21	3	75	1	1	0.4	0.2	0.1
41	Prepared	1 cup	265	81	225	9	9	5.5	2.6	0.4
	Natural									
42	Powder	4-5 heaping tsp	21	3	80	2	1	0.3	0.2	0.1
43	Prepared	1 cup	265	81	231	10	9	5.4	2.5	0.4
	Milk and milk beverages. See Dairy Products.									
44	Rice beverage, canned (RICE DREAM)	1 cup	245	89	120	Tr	2	0.2	1.3	0.3
	Soy milk. See Legumes, Nuts, and Seeds.									
	Tea									
	Brewed									
45	Black	6 fl oz	178	100	2	0	0	Tr	Tr	Tr
	Herb									
46	Chamomile	6 fl oz	178	100	2	0	0	Tr	Tr	Tr
47	Other than chamomile	6 fl oz	178	100	2	0	0	Tr	Tr	Tr
	Instant, powder, prepared									
48	Unsweetened	8 fl oz	237	100	2	0	0	0.0	0.0	0.0
49	Sweetened, lemon flavor	8 fl oz	259	91	88	Tr	0	Tr	Tr	Tr
50	Sweetened with saccharin, lemon flavor	8 fl oz	237	99	5	0	0	0.0	0.0	Tr
51	Water, tap	8 fl oz	237	100	0	0	0	0.0	0.0	0.0
	Dairy Products									
	Butter. See Fats and Oils.									
	Cheese									
	Natural									
52	Blue	1 oz	28	42	100	6	8	5.3	2.2	0.2
53	Camembert (3 wedges per 4-oz container)	1 wedge	38	52	114	8	9	5.8	2.7	0.3
	Cheddar									
54	Cut pieces	1 oz	28	37	114	7	9	6.0	2.7	0.3
55		1 cubic inch	17	37	68	4	6	3.6	1.6	0.2
56	Shredded	1 cup	113	37	455	28	37	23.8	10.6	1.1

Choles-terol (mg)	Carbo-hydrate (g)	Total dietary fiber (g)	Calcium (mg)	Iron (mg)	Potas-sium (mg)	Sodium (mg)	Vitamin A (IU)	Vitamin A (RE)	Thiamin (mg)	Ribo-flavin (mg)	Niacin (mg)	Ascor-bic acid (mg)	Food No.
						5	10	0	0.02	0.02	0.1	90	32
						55	35	2	0.05	0.06	0.1	73	33
						15	3	0	0.01	0.01	0.1	85	34
						35	88	10	0.08	0.04	0.7	115	35
						8	1,328	133	0.08	0.05	0.5	56	36
						7	52	5	0.01	0.05	Tr	10	37
						19	0	0	0.00	Tr	0.0	34	38
						7	0	0	0.00	0.00	0.0	6	39
						125	2,751	824	0.64	0.86	10.7	32	40
						244	3,058	901	0.73	1.26	10.9	34	41
						85	2,222	668	0.62	0.75	10.2	27	42
						204	2,531	742	0.71	1.14	10.4	29	43
						86	5	0	0.08	0.01	1.9	1	44
						5	0	0	0.00	0.02	0.0	0	45
						2	36	4	0.02	0.01	0.0	0	46
						2	0	0	0.02	0.01	0.0	0	47
						7	0	0	0.00	Tr	0.1	0	48
						8	0	0	0.00	0.05	0.1	0	49
						24	0	0	0.00	0.01	0.1	0	50
						7	0	0	0.00	0.00	0.0	0	51
					73	396	204	65	0.01	0.11	0.3	0	52
					71	320	351	96	0.01	0.19	0.2	0	53
					28	176	300	79	0.01	0.11	Tr	0	54
					17	105	180	47	Tr	0.06	Tr	0	55
119	1	0.0	815	0.8	111	701	1,197	314	0.03	0.42	0.1	0	56

Table 9. Nutritive Value of the Edible Part of Food

Food No.	Food Description	Measure of edible portion	Weight (g)	Water (%)	Calories (kcal)	Protein (g)	Total fat (g)	Fatty acids		
								Saturated (g)	Mono-unsaturated (g)	Poly-unsaturated (g)

Dairy Products (continued)

Cheese (continued)
Natural (continued)
Cottage
Creamed (4% fat)

Food No.	Food Description	Measure	Weight	Water	Calories	Protein	Total fat	Saturated	Mono	Poly
57	Large curd	1 cup	225	79	233	28	10	6.4	2.9	0.3
58	Small curd	1 cup	210	79	217	26	9	6.0	2.7	0.3
59	With fruit	1 cup	226	72	279	22	8	4.9	2.2	0.2
60	Low fat (2%)	1 cup	226	79	203	31	4	2.8	1.2	0.1
61	Low fat (1%)	1 cup	226	82	164	28	2	1.5	0.7	0.1
62	Uncreamed (dry curd, less than ½% fat)	1 cup	145	80	123	25	1	0.4	0.2	Tr
	Cream									
63	Regular	1 oz	28	54	99	2	10	6.2	2.8	0.4
64		1 tbsp	15	54	51	1	5	3.2	1.4	0.2
65	Low fat	1 tbsp	15	64	35	2	3	1.7	0.7	0.1
66	Fat free	1 tbsp	16	76	15	2	Tr	0.1	0.1	Tr
67	Feta	1 oz	28	55	75	4	6	4.2	1.3	0.2
68	Low fat, cheddar or colby	1 oz	28	63	49	7	2	1.2	0.6	0.1
	Mozzarella, made with									
69	Whole milk	1 oz	28	54	80	6	6	3.7	1.9	0.2
70	Part skim milk (low moisture)	1 oz	28	49	79	8	5	3.1	1.4	0.1
71	Muenster	1 oz	28	42	104	7	9	5.4	2.5	0.2
72	Neufchatel	1 oz	28	62	74	3	7	4.2	1.9	0.2
73	Parmesan, grated	1 cup	100	18	456	42	30	19.1	8.7	0.7
74		1 tbsp	5	18	23	2	2	1.0	0.4	Tr
75		1 oz	28	18	129	12	9	5.4	2.5	0.2
76	Provolone	1 oz	28	41	100	7	8	4.8	2.1	0.2
	Ricotta, made with									
77	Whole milk	1 cup	246	72	428	28	32	20.4	8.9	0.9
78	Part skim milk	1 cup	246	74	340	28	19	12.1	5.7	0.6
79	Swiss	1 oz	28	37	107	8	8	5.0	2.1	0.3
	Pasteurized process cheese									
	American									
80	Regular	1 oz	28	39	106	6	9	5.6	2.5	0.3
81	Fat free	1 slice	21	57	31	5	Tr	0.1	Tr	Tr
82	Swiss	1 oz	28	42	95	7	7	4.5	2.0	0.2
83	Pasteurized process cheese food, American	1 oz	28	43	93	6	7	4.4	2.0	0.2
84	Pasteurized process cheese spread, American	1 oz	28	48	82	5	6	3.8	1.8	0.2
	Cream, sweet									
85	Half and half (cream and milk)	1 cup	242	81	315	7	28	17.3	8.0	1.0
86		1 tbsp	15	81	20	Tr	2	1.1	0.5	0.1
87	Light, coffee, or table	1 cup	240	74	469	6	46	28.8	13.4	1.7
88		1 tbsp	15	74	29	Tr	3	1.8	0.8	0.1
	Whipping, unwhipped (volume about double when whipped)									
89	Light	1 cup	239	64	699	5	74	46.2	21.7	2.1
90		1 tbsp	15	64	44	Tr	5	2.9	1.4	0.1
91	Heavy	1 cup	238	58	821	5	88	54.8	25.4	3.3
92		1 tbsp	15	58	52	Tr	6	3.5	1.6	0.2
93	Whipped topping (pressurized)	1 cup	60	61	154	2	13	8.3	3.9	0.5
94		1 tbsp	3	61	8	Tr	1	0.4	0.2	Tr

Choles-terol (mg)	Carbo-hydrate (g)	Total dietary fiber (g)	Calcium (mg)	Iron (mg)	Potas-sium (mg)	Sodium (mg)	Vitamin A (IU)	Vitamin A (RE)	Thiamin (mg)	Ribo-flavin (mg)	Niacin (mg)	Ascor-bic acid (mg)	Food No.
34	6	0.0	135	0.3	190	911	367	108	0.05	0.37	0.3	0	57
31	6	0.0	126	0.3	177	850	342	101	0.04	0.34	0.3	0	58
25	30	0.0	108	0.2	151	915	278	81	0.04	0.29	0.2	0	59
19	8	0.0	155	0.4	217	918	158	45	0.05	0.42	0.3	0	60
10	6	0.0	138	0.3	193	918	84	25	0.05	0.37	0.3	0	61
10	3	0.0	46	0.3	47	19	44	12	0.04	0.21	0.2	0	62
31	1	0.0	23	0.3	34	84	405	108	Tr	0.06	Tr	0	63
16	Tr	0.0	12	0.2	17	43	207	55	Tr	0.03	Tr	0	64
8	1	0.0	17	0.3	25	44	108	33	Tr	0.04	Tr	0	65
1	1	0.0	29	Tr	25	85	145	44	0.01	0.03	Tr	0	66
25	1	0.0	140	0.2	18	316	127	36	0.04	0.24	0.3	0	67
6	1	0.0	118	0.1	19	174	66	18	Tr	0.06	Tr	0	68
22	1	0.0	147	0.1	19	106	225	68	Tr	0.07	Tr	0	69
15	1	0.0	207	0.1	27	150	199	54	0.01	0.10	Tr	0	70
27	Tr	0.0	203	0.1	38	178	318	90	Tr	0.09	Tr	0	71
22	1	0.0	21	0.1	32	113	321	85	Tr	0.06	Tr	0	72
79	4	0.0	1,376	1.0	107	1,862	701	173	0.05	0.39	0.3	0	73
4	Tr	0.0	69	Tr	5	93	35	9	Tr	0.02	Tr	0	74
22	1	0.0	390	0.3	30	528	199	49	0.01	0.11	0.1	0	75
20	1	0.0	214	0.1	39	248	231	75	0.01	0.09	Tr	0	76
124	7	0.0	509	0.9	257	207	1,205	330	0.03	0.48	0.3	0	77
76	13	0.0	669	1.1	308	307	1,063	278	0.05	0.46	0.2	0	78
26	1	0.0	272	Tr	31	74	240	72	0.01	0.10	Tr	0	79
27	Tr	0.0	174	0.1	46	406	343	82	0.01	0.10	Tr	0	80
2	3	0.0	145	0.1	60	321	308	92	0.01	0.10	Tr	0	81
24	1	0.0	219	0.2	61	388	229	65	Tr	0.08	Tr	0	82
18	2	0.0	163	0.2	79	337	259	62	0.01	0.13	Tr	0	83
16	2	0.0	159	0.1	69	381	223	54	0.01	0.12	Tr	0	84
89	10	0.0	254	0.2	314	98	1,050	259	0.08	0.36	0.2	2	85
6	1	0.0	16	Tr	19	6	65	16	0.01	0.02	Tr	Tr	86
159	9	0.0	231	0.1	292	95	1,519	437	0.08	0.36	0.1	2	87
10	1	0.0	14	Tr	18	6	95	27	Tr	0.02	Tr	Tr	88
265	7	0.0	166	0.1	231	82	2,694	705	0.06	0.30	0.1	1	89
17	Tr	0.0	10	Tr	15	5	169	44	Tr	0.02	Tr	Tr	90
326	7	0.0	154	0.1	179	89	3,499	1,002	0.05	0.26	0.1	1	91
21	Tr	0.0	10	Tr	11	6	221	63	Tr	0.02	Tr	Tr	92
46	7	0.0	61	Tr	88	78	506	124	0.02	0.04	Tr	0	93
2	Tr	0.0	3	Tr	4	4	25	6	Tr	Tr	Tr	0	94

Table 9. Nutritive Value of the Edible Part of Food

Food No.	Food Description	Measure of edible portion	Weight (g)	Water (%)	Calories (kcal)	Protein (g)	Total fat (g)	Fatty acids Saturated (g)	Mono-unsaturated (g)	Poly-unsaturated (g)
	Dairy Products (continued)									
	Cream, sour									
95	Regular	1 cup	230	71	493	7	48	30.0	13.9	1.8
96		1 tbsp	12	71	26	Tr	3	1.6	0.7	0.1
97	Reduced fat	1 tbsp	15	80	20	Tr	2	1.1	0.5	0.1
98	Fat free	1 tbsp	16	81	12	Tr	0	0.0	0.0	0.0
	Cream product, imitation (made with vegetable fat)									
	Sweet									
	Creamer									
99	Liquid (frozen)	1 tbsp	15	77	20	Tr	1	0.3	1.1	Tr
100	Powdered	1 tsp	2	2	11	Tr	1	0.7	Tr	Tr
	Whipped topping									
101	Frozen	1 cup	75	50	239	1	19	16.3	1.2	0.4
102		1 tbsp	4	50	13	Tr	1	0.9	0.1	Tr
103	Powdered, prepared with whole milk	1 cup	80	67	151	3	10	8.5	0.7	0.2
104		1 tbsp	4	67	8	Tr	Tr	0.4	Tr	Tr
105	Pressurized	1 cup	70	60	184	1	16	13.2	1.3	0.2
106		1 tbsp	4	60	11	Tr	1	0.8	0.1	Tr
107	Sour dressing (filled cream type, nonbutterfat)	1 cup	235	75	417	8	39	31.2	4.6	1.1
108		1 tbsp	12	75	21	Tr	2	1.6	0.2	0.1
	Frozen dessert									
	Frozen yogurt, soft serve									
109	Chocolate	½ cup	72	64	115	3	4	2.6	1.3	0.2
110	Vanilla	½ cup	72	65	114	3	4	2.5	1.1	0.2
	Ice cream									
	Regular									
111	Chocolate	½ cup	66	56	143	3	7	4.5	2.1	0.3
112	Vanilla	½ cup	66	61	133	2	7	4.5	2.1	0.3
113	Light (50% reduced fat), vanilla	½ cup	66	68	92	3	3	1.7	0.8	0.1
114	Premium low fat, chocolate	½ cup	72	61	113	3	2	1.0	0.6	0.1
115	Rich, vanilla	½ cup	74	57	178	3	12	7.4	3.4	0.4
116	Soft serve, french vanilla	½ cup	86	60	185	4	11	6.4	3.0	0.4
117	Sherbet, orange	½ cup	74	66	102	1	1	0.9	0.4	0.1
	Milk									
	Fluid, no milk solids added									
118	Whole (3.3% fat)	1 cup	244	88	150	8	8	5.1	2.4	0.3
119	Reduced fat (2%)	1 cup	244	89	121	8	5	2.9	1.4	0.2
120	Lowfat (1%)	1 cup	244	90	102	8	3	1.6	0.7	0.1
121	Nonfat (skim)	1 cup	245	91	86	8	Tr	0.3	0.1	Tr
122	Buttermilk	1 cup	245	90	99	8	2	1.3	0.6	0.1
	Canned									
123	Condensed, sweetened	1 cup	306	27	982	24	27	16.8	7.4	1.0
	Evaporated									
124	Whole milk	1 cup	252	74	339	17	19	11.6	5.9	0.6
125	Skim milk	1 cup	256	79	199	19	1	0.3	0.2	Tr
	Dried									
126	Buttermilk	1 cup	120	3	464	41	7	4.3	2.0	0.3
127	Nonfat, instant, with added vitamin A	1 cup	68	4	244	24	Tr	0.3	0.1	Tr
	Milk beverage									
	Chocolate milk (commercial)									
128	Whole	1 cup	250	82	208	8	8	5.3	2.5	0.3
129	Reduced fat (2%)	1 cup	250	84	179	8	5	3.1	1.5	0.2
130	Lowfat (1%)	1 cup	250	85	158	8	3	1.5	0.8	0.1

*The vitamin A values listed for imitation sweet cream products are mostly from beta-carotene added for coloring.

Choles-terol (mg)	Carbo-hydrate (g)	Total dietary fiber (g)	Calcium (mg)	Iron (mg)	Potas-sium (mg)	Sodium (mg)	Vitamin A (IU)	Vitamin A (RE)	Thiamin (mg)	Ribo-flavin (mg)	Niacin (mg)	Ascor-bic acid (mg)	Food No.
102	10	0.0	268	0.1	331	123	1,817	449	0.08	0.34	0.2	2	95
5	1	0.0	14	Tr	17	6	95	23	Tr	0.02	Tr	Tr	96
6	1	0.0	16	Tr	19	6	68	17	0.01	0.02	Tr	Tr	97
1	2	0.0	20	0.0	21	23	100	13	0.01	0.02	Tr	0	98
0	2	0.0	1	Tr	29	12	13*	1*	0.00	0.00	0.0	0	99
0	1	0.0	Tr	Tr	16	4	4	Tr	0.00	Tr	0.0	0	100
0	17	0.0	5	0.1	14	19	646*	65*	0.00	0.00	0.0	0	101
0	1	0.0	Tr	Tr	1	1	34*	3*	0.00	0.00	0.0	0	102
8	13	0.0	72	Tr	121	53	289*	39*	0.02	0.09	Tr	1	103
Tr	1	0.0	4	Tr	6	3	14*	2*	Tr	Tr	Tr	Tr	104
0	11	0.0	4	Tr	13	43	331*	33*	0.00	0.00	0.0	0	105
0	1	0.0	Tr	Tr	1	2	19*	2*	0.00	0.00	0.0	0	106
13	11	0.0	266	0.1	380	113	24	5	0.09	0.38	0.2	2	107
1	1	0.0	14	Tr	19	6	1	Tr	Tr	0.02	Tr	Tr	108
4	18	1.6	106	0.9	188	71	115	31	0.03	0.15	0.2	Tr	109
1	17	0.0	103	0.2	152	63	153	41	0.03	0.16	0.2	1	110
22	19	0.8	72	0.6	164	50	275	79	0.03	0.13	0.1	Tr	111
29	16	0.0	84	0.1	131	53	270	77	0.03	0.16	0.1	Tr	112
9	15	0.0	92	0.1	139	56	109	31	0.04	0.17	0.1	1	113
7	22	0.7	107	0.4	179	50	163	47	0.02	0.13	0.1	1	114
45	17	0.0	87	Tr	118	41	476	136	0.03	0.12	0.1	1	115
78	19	0.0	113	0.2	152	52	464	132	0.04	0.16	0.1	1	116
4	22	0.0	40	0.1	71	34	56	10	0.02	0.06	Tr	2	117
33	11	0.0	291	0.1	370	120	307	76	0.09	0.40	0.2	2	118
18	12	0.0	297	0.1	377	122	500	139	0.10	0.40	0.2	2	119
10	12	0.0	300	0.1	381	123	500	144	0.10	0.41	0.2	2	120
4	12	0.0	302	0.1	406	126	500	149	0.09	0.34	0.2	2	121
9	12	0.0	285	0.1	371	257	81	20	0.08	0.38	0.1	2	122
104	166	0.0	868	0.6	1,136	389	1,004	248	0.28	1.27	0.6	8	123
74	25	0.0	657	0.5	764	267	612	136	0.12	0.80	0.5	5	124
9	29	0.0	741	0.7	849	294	1,004	300	0.12	0.79	0.4	3	125
83	59	0.0	1,421	0.4	1,910	621	262	65	0.47	1.89	1.1	7	126
12	35	0.0	837	0.2	1,160	373	1,612	483	0.28	1.19	0.6	4	127
31	26	2.0	280	0.6	417	149	303	73	0.09	0.41	0.3	2	128
17	26	1.3	284	0.6	422	151	500	143	0.09	0.41	0.3	2	129
7	26	1.3	287	0.6	426	152	500	148	0.10	0.42	0.3	2	130

Table 9. Nutritive Value of the Edible Part of Food

Food No.	Food Description	Measure of edible portion	Weight (g)	Water (%)	Calories (kcal)	Protein (g)	Total fat (g)	Fatty acids Saturated (g)	Fatty acids Mono-unsaturated (g)	Fatty acids Poly-unsaturated (g)
	Dairy Products (continued)									
	Milk beverage (continued)									
131	Eggnog (commercial)	1 cup	254	74	342	10	19	11.3	5.7	0.9
	Milk shake, thick									
132	Chocolate	10.6 fl oz	300	72	356	9	8	5.0	2.3	0.3
133	Vanilla	11 fl oz	313	74	350	12	9	5.9	2.7	0.4
	Sherbet. See Dairy Products, frozen dessert.									
	Yogurt									
	With added milk solids									
	Made with lowfat milk									
134	Fruit flavored	8-oz container	227	74	231	10	2	1.6	0.7	0.1
135	Plain	8-oz container	227	85	144	12	4	2.3	1.0	0.1
	Made with nonfat milk									
136	Fruit flavored	8-oz container	227	75	213	10	Tr	0.3	0.1	Tr
137	Plain	8-oz container	227	85	127	13	Tr	0.3	0.1	Tr
	Without added milk solids									
138	Made with whole milk, plain	8-oz container	227	88	139	8	7	4.8	2.0	0.2
139	Made with nonfat milk, low calorie sweetener, vanilla or lemon flavor	8-oz container	227	87	98	9	Tr	0.3	0.1	Tr
	Eggs									
	Egg									
	Raw									
140	Whole	1 medium	44	75	66	5	4	1.4	1.7	0.6
141		1 large	50	75	75	6	5	1.6	1.9	0.7
142		1 extra large	58	75	86	7	6	1.8	2.2	0.8
143	White	1 large	33	88	17	4	0	0.0	0.0	0.0
144	Yolk	1 large	17	49	59	3	5	1.6	1.9	0.7
	Cooked, whole									
145	Fried, in margarine, with salt	1 large	46	69	92	6	7	1.9	2.7	1.3
146	Hard cooked, shell removed	1 large	50	75	78	6	5	1.6	2.0	0.7
147		1 cup, chopped	136	75	211	17	14	4.4	5.5	1.9
148	Poached, with salt	1 large	50	75	75	6	5	1.5	1.9	0.7
149	Scrambled, in margarine, with whole milk, salt	1 large	61	73	101	7	7	2.2	2.9	1.3
150	Egg substitute, liquid	¼ cup	63	83	53	8	2	0.4	0.6	1.0
	Fats and Oils									
	Butter (4 sticks per lb)									
151	Salted	1 stick	113	16	813	1	92	57.3	26.6	3.4
152		1 tbsp	14	16	102	Tr	12	7.2	3.3	0.4
153		1 tsp	5	16	36	Tr	4	2.5	1.2	0.2
154	Unsalted	1 stick	113	18	813	1	92	57.3	26.6	3.4
155	Lard	1 cup	205	0	1,849	0	205	80.4	92.5	23.0
156		1 tbsp	13	0	115	0	13	5.0	5.8	1.4
	Margarine, vitamin A-fortified, salt added									
	Regular (about 80% fat)									
157	Hard (4 sticks per lb)	1 stick	113	16	815	1	91	17.9	40.6	28.8
158		1 tbsp	14	16	101	Tr	11	2.2	5.0	3.6
159		1 tsp	5	16	34	Tr	4	0.7	1.7	1.2
160	Soft	1 cup	227	16	1,626	2	183	31.3	64.7	78.5
161		1 tsp	5	16	34	Tr	4	0.6	1.3	1.6

Choles-terol (mg)	Carbo-hydrate (g)	Total dietary fiber (g)	Calcium (mg)	Iron (mg)	Potas-sium (mg)	Sodium (mg)	Vitamin A		Thiamin (mg)	Ribo-flavin (mg)	Niacin (mg)	Ascor-bic acid (mg)	Food No.
							(IU)	(RE)					
149	34	0.0	330	0.5	420	138	894	203	0.09	0.48	0.3	4	131
32	63	0.9	396	0.9	672	333	258	63	0.14	0.67	0.4	0	132
37	56	0.0	457	0.3	572	299	357	88	0.09	0.61	0.5	0	133
10	43	0.0	345	0.2	442	133	104	25	0.08	0.40	0.2	1	134
14	16	0.0	415	0.2	531	159	150	36	0.10	0.49	0.3	2	135
5	43	0.0	345	0.2	440	132	16	5	0.09	0.41	0.2	2	136
4	17	0.0	452	0.2	579	174	16	5	0.11	0.53	0.3	2	137
29	11	0.0	274	0.1	351	105	279	68	0.07	0.32	0.2	1	138
5	17	0.0	325	0.3	402	134	0	0	0.08	0.37	0.2	2	139
187	1	0.0	22	0.6	53	55	279	84	0.03	0.22	Tr	0	140
213	1	0.0	25	0.7	61	63	318	96	0.03	0.25	Tr	0	141
247	1	0.0	28	0.8	70	73	368	111	0.04	0.29	Tr	0	142
0	Tr	0.0	2	Tr	48	55	0	0	Tr	0.15	Tr	0	143
213	Tr	0.0	23	0.6	16	7	323	97	0.03	0.11	Tr	0	144
211	1	0.0	25	0.7	61	162	394	114	0.03	0.24	Tr	0	145
212	1	0.0	25	0.6	63	62	280	84	0.03	0.26	Tr	0	146
577	2	0.0	68	1.6	171	169	762	228	0.09	0.70	0.1	0	147
212	1	0.0	25	0.7	60	140	316	95	0.02	0.22	Tr	0	148
215	1	0.0	43	0.7	84	171	416	119	0.03	0.27	Tr	Tr	149
1	Tr	0.0	33	1.3	208	112	1,361	136	0.07	0.19	0.1	0	150
248	Tr	0.0	27	0.2	29	937	3,468	855	0.01	0.04	Tr	0	151
31	Tr	0.0	3	Tr	4	117	434	107	Tr	Tr	Tr	0	152
11	Tr	0.0	1	Tr	1	41	153	38	Tr	Tr	Tr	0	153
248	Tr	0.0	27	0.2	29	12	3,468	855	0.01	0.04	Tr	0	154
195	0	0.0	Tr	0.0	Tr	Tr	0	0	0.00	0.00	0.0	0	155
12	0	0.0	Tr	0.0	Tr	Tr	0	0	0.00	0.00	0.0	0	156
0	1	0.0	34	0.1	48	1,070	4,050	906	0.01	0.04	Tr	Tr	157
0	Tr	0.0	4	Tr	6	132	500	112	Tr	0.01	Tr	Tr	158
0	Tr	0.0	1	Tr	2	44	168	38	Tr	Tr	Tr	Tr	159
0	1	0.0	60	0.0	86	2,449	8,106	1,814	0.02	0.07	Tr	Tr	160
0	Tr	0.0	1	0.0	2	51	168	38	Tr	Tr	Tr	Tr	161

Table 9. Nutritive Value of the Edible Part of Food

Food No.	Food Description	Measure of edible portion	Weight (g)	Water (%)	Calories (kcal)	Protein (g)	Total fat (g)	Fatty acids Saturated (g)	Mono-unsaturated (g)	Poly-unsaturated (g)
	Fats and Oils (continued)									
	Margarine, vitamin A-fortified, salt added (continued)									
	Spread (about 60% fat)									
162	Hard (4 sticks per lb)	1 stick	115	37	621	1	70	16.2	29.9	20.8
163		1 tbsp	14	37	76	Tr	9	2.0	3.6	2.5
164		1 tsp	5	37	26	Tr	3	0.7	1.2	0.9
165	Soft	1 cup	229	37	1,236	1	139	29.3	72.1	31.6
166		1 tsp	5	37	26	Tr	3	0.6	1.5	0.7
167	Spread (about 40% fat)	1 cup	232	58	801	1	90	17.9	36.4	32.0
168		1 tsp	5	58	17	Tr	2	0.4	0.8	0.7
169	Margarine butter blend	1 stick	113	16	811	1	91	32.1	37.0	18.0
170		1 tbsp	14	16	102	Tr	11	4.0	4.7	2.3
	Oils, salad or cooking									
171	Canola	1 cup	218	0	1,927	0	218	15.5	128.4	64.5
172		1 tbsp	14	0	124	0	14	1.0	8.2	4.1
173	Corn	1 cup	218	0	1,927	0	218	27.7	52.8	128.0
174		1 tbsp	14	0	120	0	14	1.7	3.3	8.0
175	Olive	1 cup	216	0	1,909	0	216	29.2	159.2	18.1
176		1 tbsp	14	0	119	0	14	1.8	9.9	1.1
177	Peanut	1 cup	216	0	1,909	0	216	36.5	99.8	69.1
178		1 tbsp	14	0	119	0	14	2.3	6.2	4.3
179	Safflower, high oleic	1 cup	218	0	1,927	0	218	13.5	162.7	31.3
180		1 tbsp	14	0	120	0	14	0.8	10.2	2.0
181	Sesame	1 cup	218	0	1,927	0	218	31.0	86.5	90.9
182		1 tbsp	14	0	120	0	14	1.9	5.4	5.7
183	Soybean, hydrogenated	1 cup	218	0	1,927	0	218	32.5	93.7	82.0
184		1 tbsp	14	0	120	0	14	2.0	5.8	5.1
185	Soybean, hydrogenated and cottonseed oil blend	1 cup	218	0	1,927	0	218	39.2	64.3	104.9
186		1 tbsp	14	0	120	0	14	2.4	4.0	6.5
187	Sunflower	1 cup	218	0	1,927	0	218	22.5	42.5	143.2
188		1 tbsp	14	0	120	0	14	1.4	2.7	8.9
	Salad dressings									
	Commercial									
	Blue cheese									
189	Regular	1 tbsp	15	32	77	1	8	1.5	1.9	4.3
190	Low calorie	1 tbsp	15	80	15	1	1	0.4	0.3	0.4
	Caesar									
191	Regular	1 tbsp	15	34	78	Tr	8	1.3	2.0	4.8
192	Low calorie	1 tbsp	15	73	17	Tr	1	0.1	0.2	0.4
	French									
193	Regular	1 tbsp	16	38	67	Tr	6	1.5	1.2	3.4
194	Low calorie	1 tbsp	16	69	22	Tr	1	0.1	0.2	0.6
	Italian									
195	Regular	1 tbsp	15	38	69	Tr	7	1.0	1.6	4.1
196	Low calorie	1 tbsp	15	82	16	Tr	1	0.2	0.3	0.9
	Mayonnaise									
197	Regular	1 tbsp	14	15	99	Tr	11	1.6	3.1	5.7
198	Light, cholesterol free	1 tbsp	15	56	49	Tr	5	0.7	1.1	2.8
199	Fat free	1 tbsp	16	84	12	0	Tr	0.1	0.1	0.2
	Russian									
200	Regular	1 tbsp	15	35	76	Tr	8	1.1	1.8	4.5
201	Low calorie	1 tbsp	16	65	23	Tr	1	0.1	0.1	0.4
	Thousand island									
202	Regular	1 tbsp	16	46	59	Tr	6	0.9	1.3	3.1
203	Low calorie	1 tbsp	15	69	24	Tr	2	0.2	0.4	0.9

Choles-terol (mg)	Carbo-hydrate (g)	Total dietary fiber (g)	Calcium (mg)	Iron (mg)	Potas-sium (mg)	Sodium (mg)	Vitamin A (IU)	Vitamin A (RE)	Thiamin (mg)	Ribo-flavin (mg)	Niacin (mg)	Ascor-bic acid (mg)	Food No.
0	0	0.0	24	0.0	34	1,143	4,107	919	0.01	0.03	Tr	Tr	162
0	0	0.0	3	0.0	4	139	500	112	Tr	Tr	Tr	Tr	163
0	0	0.0	1	0.0	1	48	171	38	Tr	Tr	Tr	Tr	164
0	0	0.0	48	0.0	68	2,276	8,178	1,830	0.02	0.06	Tr	Tr	165
0	0	0.0	1	0.0	1	48	171	38	Tr	Tr	Tr	Tr	166
0	1	0.0	41	0.0	59	2,226	8,285	1,854	0.01	0.05	Tr	Tr	167
0	Tr	0.0	1	0.0	1	46	171	38	Tr	Tr	Tr	Tr	168
99	1	0.0	32	0.1	41	1,014	4,035	903	0.01	0.04	Tr	Tr	169
12	Tr	0.0	4	Tr	5	127	507	113	Tr	Tr	Tr	Tr	170
0	0	0.0	0	0.0	0	0	0	0	0.00	0.00	0.0	0	171
0	0	0.0	0	0.0	0	0	0	0	0.00	0.00	0.0	0	172
0	0	0.0	0	0.0	0	0	0	0	0.00	0.00	0.0	0	173
0	0	0.0	0	0.0	0	0	0	0	0.00	0.00	0.0	0	174
0	0	0.0	Tr	0.8	0	Tr	0	0	0.00	0.00	0.0	0	175
0	0	0.0	Tr	0.1	0	Tr	0	0	0.00	0.00	0.0	0	176
0	0	0.0	Tr	0.1	Tr	Tr	0	0	0.00	0.00	0.0	0	177
0	0	0.0	Tr	Tr	Tr	Tr	0	0	0.00	0.00	0.0	0	178
0	0	0.0	0	0.0	0	0	0	0	0.00	0.00	0.0	0	179
0	0	0.0	0	0.0	0	0	0	0	0.00	0.00	0.0	0	180
0	0	0.0	0	0.0	0	0	0	0	0.00	0.00	0.0	0	181
0	0	0.0	0	0.0	0	0	0	0	0.00	0.00	0.0	0	182
0	0	0.0	0	0.0	0	0	0	0	0.00	0.00	0.0	0	183
0	0	0.0	0	0.0	0	0	0	0	0.00	0.00	0.0	0	184
0	0	0.0	0	0.0	0	0	0	0	0.00	0.00	0.0	0	185
0	0	0.0	0	0.0	0	0	0	0	0.00	0.00	0.0	0	186
0	0	0.0	0	0.0	0	0	0	0	0.00	0.00	0.0	0	187
0	0	0.0	0	0.0	0	0	0	0	0.00	0.00	0.0	0	188
3	1	0.0	12	Tr	6	167	32	10	Tr	0.02	Tr	Tr	189
Tr	Tr	0.0	14	0.1	1	184	2	Tr	Tr	0.02	Tr	Tr	190
Tr	Tr	Tr	4	Tr	4	158	3	Tr	Tr	Tr	Tr	0	191
Tr	3	Tr	4	Tr	4	162	3	Tr	Tr	Tr	Tr	0	192
0	3	0.0	2	0.1	12	214	203	20	Tr	Tr	Tr	0	193
0	4	0.0	2	0.1	13	128	212	21	0.00	0.00	0.0	0	194
0	1	0.0	1	Tr	2	116	11	4	Tr	Tr	Tr	0	195
1	1	Tr	Tr	Tr	2	118	0	0	0.00	0.00	0.0	0	196
8	Tr	0.0	2	0.1	5	78	39	12	0.00	0.00	Tr	0	197
0	1	0.0	0	0.0	10	107	18	2	0.00	0.00	0.0	0	198
0	2	0.6	0	0.0	15	190	0	0	0.00	0.00	0.0	0	199
3	2	0.0	3	0.1	24	133	106	32	0.01	0.01	0.1	1	200
1	4	Tr	3	0.1	26	141	9	3	Tr	Tr	Tr	1	201
4	2	0.0	2	0.1	18	109	50	15	Tr	Tr	Tr	0	202
2	2	0.2	2	0.1	17	153	49	15	Tr	Tr	Tr	0	203

Table 9. Nutritive Value of the Edible Part of Food

Food No.	Food Description	Measure of edible portion	Weight (g)	Water (%)	Calories (kcal)	Protein (g)	Total fat (g)	Fatty acids Saturated (g)	Mono-unsaturated (g)	Poly-unsaturated (g)
	Fats and Oils (continued)									
	Salad dressings (continued)									
	Prepared from home recipe									
204	Cooked, made with margarine	1 tbsp	16	69	25	1	2	0.5	0.6	0.3
205	French	1 tbsp	14	24	88	Tr	10	1.8	2.9	4.7
206	Vinegar and oil	1 tbsp	16	47	70	0	8	1.4	2.3	3.8
207	Shortening (hydrogenated soybean and cottonseed oils)	1 cup	205	0	1,812	0	205	51.3	91.2	53.5
208		1 tbsp	13	0	113	0	13	3.2	5.7	3.3
	Fish and Shellfish									
209	Catfish, breaded, fried	3 oz	85	59	195	15	11	2.8	4.8	2.8
	Clam									
210	Raw, meat only	3 oz	85	82	63	11	1	0.1	0.1	0.2
211		1 medium	15	82	11	2	Tr	Tr	Tr	Tr
212	Breaded, fried	¾ cup	115	29	451	13	26	6.6	11.4	6.8
213	Canned, drained solids	3 oz	85	64	126	22	2	0.2	0.1	0.5
214		1 cup	160	64	237	41	3	0.3	0.3	0.9
	Cod									
215	Baked or broiled	3 oz	85	76	89	20	1	0.1	0.1	0.3
216		1 fillet	90	76	95	21	1	0.1	0.1	0.3
217	Canned, solids and liquid	3 oz	85	76	89	19	1	0.1	0.1	0.2
	Crab									
	Alaska king									
218	Steamed	1 leg	134	78	130	26	2	0.2	0.2	0.7
219		3 oz	85	78	82	16	1	0.1	0.2	0.5
220	Imitation, from surimi	3 oz	85	74	87	10	1	0.2	0.2	0.6
	Blue									
221	Steamed	3 oz	85	77	87	17	2	0.2	0.2	0.6
222	Canned crabmeat	1 cup	135	76	134	28	2	0.3	0.3	0.6
223	Crab cake, with egg, onion, fried in margarine	1 cake	60	71	93	12	5	0.9	1.7	1.4
224	Fish fillet, battered or breaded, fried	1 fillet	91	54	211	13	11	2.6	2.3	5.7
225	Fish stick and portion, breaded, frozen, reheated	1 stick (4" x 1" x ½")	28	46	76	4	3	0.9	1.4	0.9
226		1 portion (4" x 2" x ½")	57	46	155	9	7	1.8	2.9	1.8
227	Flounder or sole, baked or broiled	3 oz	85	73	99	21	1	0.3	0.2	0.5
228		1 fillet	127	73	149	31	2	0.5	0.3	0.8
229	Haddock, baked or broiled	3 oz	85	74	95	21	1	0.1	0.1	0.3
230		1 fillet	150	74	168	36	1	0.3	0.2	0.5
231	Halibut, baked or broiled	3 oz	85	72	119	23	2	0.4	0.8	0.8
232		½ fillet	159	72	223	42	5	0.7	1.5	1.5
233	Herring, pickled	3 oz	85	55	223	12	15	2.0	10.2	1.4
234	Lobster, steamed	3 oz	85	76	83	17	1	0.1	0.1	0.1
235	Ocean perch, baked or broiled	3 oz	85	73	103	20	2	0.3	0.7	0.5
236		1 fillet	50	73	61	12	1	0.2	0.4	0.3
	Oyster									
237	Raw, meat only	1 cup	248	85	169	17	6	1.9	0.8	2.4
238		6 medium	84	85	57	6	2	0.6	0.3	0.8
239	Breaded, fried	3 oz	85	65	167	7	11	2.7	4.0	2.8
240	Pollock, baked or broiled	3 oz	85	74	96	20	1	0.2	0.1	0.4
241		1 fillet	60	74	68	14	1	0.1	0.1	0.3
242	Rockfish, baked or broiled	3 oz	85	73	103	20	2	0.4	0.4	0.5
243		1 fillet	149	73	180	36	3	0.7	0.7	0.9

Choles-terol (mg)	Carbo-hydrate (g)	Total dietary fiber (g)	Calcium (mg)	Iron (mg)	Potas-sium (mg)	Sodium (mg)	Vitamin A		Thiamin (mg)	Ribo-flavin (mg)	Niacin (mg)	Ascor-bic acid (mg)	Food No.
							(IU)	(RE)					
9	2	0.0	13	0.1	19	117	66	20	0.01	0.02	Tr	Tr	204
0	Tr	0.0	1	Tr	3	92	72	22	Tr	Tr	Tr	Tr	205
0	Tr	0.0	0	0.0	1	Tr	0	0	0.00	0.00	0.0	0	206
0	0	0.0	0	0.0	0	0	0	0	0.00	0.00	0.0	0	207
0	0	0.0	0	0.0	0	0	0	0	0.00	0.00	0.0	0	208
69	7	0.6	37	1.2	289	238	24	7	0.06	0.11	1.9	0	209
29	2	0.0	39	11.9	267	48	255	77	0.07	0.18	1.5	11	210
5	Tr	0.0	7	2.0	46	8	44	13	0.01	0.03	0.3	2	211
87	39	0.3	21	3.0	266	834	122	37	0.21	0.26	2.9	0	212
57	4	0.0	78	23.8	534	95	485	145	0.13	0.36	2.9	19	213
107	8	0.0	147	44.7	1,005	179	912	274	0.24	0.68	5.4	35	214
40	0	0.0	8	0.3	439	77	27	9	0.02	0.04	2.1	3	215
42	0	0.0	8	0.3	465	82	29	9	0.02	0.05	2.2	3	216
47	0	0.0	18	0.4	449	185	39	12	0.07	0.07	2.1	1	217
71	0	0.0	79	1.0	351	1,436	39	12	0.07	0.07	1.8	10	218
45	0	0.0	50	0.6	223	911	25	8	0.05	0.05	1.1	6	219
17	9	0.0	11	0.3	77	715	56	17	0.03	0.02	0.2	0	220
85	0	0.0	88	0.8	275	237	5	2	0.09	0.04	2.8	3	221
120	0	0.0	136	1.1	505	450	7	3	0.11	0.11	1.8	4	222
90	Tr	0.0	63	0.6	194	198	151	49	0.05	0.05	1.7	2	223
31	15	0.5	16	1.9	291	484	35	11	0.10	0.10	1.9	0	224
31	7	0.0	6	0.2	73	163	30	9	0.04	0.05	0.6	0	225
64	14	0.0	11	0.4	149	332	60	18	0.07	0.10	1.2	0	226
58	0	0.0	15	0.3	292	89	32	9	0.07	0.10	1.9	0	227
86	0	0.0	23	0.4	437	133	48	14	0.10	0.14	2.8	0	228
63	0	0.0	36	1.1	339	74	54	16	0.03	0.04	3.9	0	229
111	0	0.0	63	2.0	599	131	95	29	0.06	0.07	6.9	0	230
35	0	0.0	51	0.9	490	59	152	46	0.06	0.08	6.1	0	231
65	0	0.0	95	1.7	916	110	285	86	0.11	0.14	11.3	0	232
11	8	0.0	65	1.0	59	740	732	219	0.03	0.12	2.8	0	233
61	1	0.0	52	0.3	299	323	74	22	0.01	0.06	0.9	0	234
46	0	0.0	116	1.0	298	82	39	12	0.11	0.11	2.1	1	235
27	0	0.0	69	0.6	175	48	23	7	0.07	0.07	1.2	Tr	236
131	10	0.0	112	16.5	387	523	248	74	0.25	0.24	3.4	9	237
45	3	0.0	38	5.6	131	177	84	25	0.08	0.08	1.2	3	238
69	10	0.2	53	5.9	207	354	257	77	0.13	0.17	1.4	3	239
82	0	0.0	5	0.2	329	99	65	20	0.06	0.06	1.4	0	240
58	0	0.0	4	0.2	232	70	46	14	0.04	0.05	1.0	0	241
37	0	0.0	10	0.5	442	65	186	56	0.04	0.07	3.3	0	242
66	0	0.0	18	0.8	775	115	326	98	0.07	0.13	5.8	0	243

Table 9. Nutritive Value of the Edible Part of Food

Food No.	Food Description	Measure of edible portion	Weight (g)	Water (%)	Calories (kcal)	Protein (g)	Total fat (g)	Fatty acids Saturated (g)	Mono-unsaturated (g)	Poly-unsaturated (g)
	Fish and Shellfish (continued)									
244	Roughy, orange, baked or broiled	3 oz	85	69	76	16	1	Tr	0.5	Tr
	Salmon									
245	Baked or broiled (red)	3 oz	85	62	184	23	9	1.6	4.5	2.0
246		½ fillet	155	62	335	42	17	3.0	8.2	3.7
247	Canned (pink), solids and liquid (includes bones)	3 oz	85	69	118	17	5	1.3	1.5	1.7
248	Smoked (chinook)	3 oz	85	72	99	16	4	0.8	1.7	0.8
249	Sardine, Atlantic, canned in oil, drained solids (includes bones)	3 oz	85	60	177	21	10	1.3	3.3	4.4
	Scallop, cooked									
250	Breaded, fried	6 large	93	58	200	17	10	2.5	4.2	2.7
251	Steamed	3 oz	85	73	95	20	1	0.1	0.1	0.4
	Shrimp									
252	Breaded, fried	3 oz	85	53	206	18	10	1.8	3.2	4.3
253		6 large	45	53	109	10	6	0.9	1.7	2.3
254	Canned, drained solids	3 oz	85	73	102	20	2	0.3	0.2	0.6
255	Swordfish, baked or broiled	3 oz	85	69	132	22	4	1.2	1.7	1.0
256		1 piece	106	69	164	27	5	1.5	2.1	1.3
257	Trout, baked or broiled	3 oz	85	68	144	21	6	1.8	1.8	2.0
258		1 fillet	71	68	120	17	5	1.5	1.5	1.7
	Tuna									
259	Baked or broiled	3 oz	85	63	118	25	1	0.3	0.2	0.3
	Canned, drained solids									
260	Oil pack, chunk light	3 oz	85	60	168	25	7	1.3	2.5	2.5
261	Water pack, chunk light	3 oz	85	75	99	22	1	0.2	0.1	0.3
262	Water pack, solid white	3 oz	85	73	109	20	3	0.7	0.7	0.9
263	Tuna salad: light tuna in oil, pickle relish, mayo type salad dressing	1 cup	205	63	383	33	19	3.2	5.9	8.5
	Fruits and Fruit Juices									
	Apples									
	Raw									
264	Unpeeled, 2¾" dia (about 3 per lb)	1 apple	138	84	81	Tr	Tr	0.1	Tr	0.1
265	Peeled, sliced	1 cup	110	84	63	Tr	Tr	0.1	Tr	0.1
266	Dried (sodium bisulfite used to preserve color)	5 rings	32	32	78	Tr	Tr	Tr	Tr	Tr
267	Apple juice, bottled or canned	1 cup	248	88	117	Tr	Tr	Tr	Tr	0.1
268	Apple pie filling, canned	⅛ of 21-oz can	74	73	75	Tr	Tr	Tr	0.0	Tr
	Applesauce, canned									
269	Sweetened	1 cup	255	80	194	Tr	Tr	0.1	Tr	0.1
270	Unsweetened	1 cup	244	88	105	Tr	Tr	Tr	Tr	Tr
	Apricots									
271	Raw, without pits (about 12 per lb with pits)	1 apricot	35	86	17	Tr	Tr	Tr	0.1	Tr
	Canned, halves, fruit and liquid									
272	Heavy syrup pack	1 cup	258	78	214	1	Tr	Tr	0.1	Tr
273	Juice pack	1 cup	244	87	117	2	Tr	Tr	Tr	Tr
274	Dried, sulfured	10 halves	35	31	83	1	Tr	Tr	0.1	Tr
275	Apricot nectar, canned, with added ascorbic acid	1 cup	251	85	141	1	Tr	Tr	0.1	Tr
	Asian pear, raw									
276	2¼" high x 2½" dia	1 pear	122	88	51	1	Tr	Tr	0.1	0.1
277	3⅜" high x 3" dia	1 pear	275	88	116	1	1	Tr	0.1	0.2

Choles-terol (mg)	Carbo-hydrate (g)	Total dietary fiber (g)	Calcium (mg)	Iron (mg)	Potas-sium (mg)	Sodium (mg)	Vitamin A		Thiamin (mg)	Ribo-flavin (mg)	Niacin (mg)	Ascor-bic acid (mg)	Food No.
							(IU)	(RE)					
22	0	0.0	32	0.2	327	69	69	20	0.10	0.16	3.1	0	244
74	0	0.0	6	0.5	319	56	178	54	0.18	0.15	5.7	0	245
135	0	0.0	11	0.9	581	102	324	98	0.33	0.27	10.3	0	246
47	0	0.0	181	0.7	277	471	47	14	0.02	0.16	5.6	0	247
20	0	0.0	9	0.7	149	666	75	22	0.02	0.09	4.0	0	248
121	0	0.0	325	2.5	337	429	190	57	0.07	0.19	4.5	0	249
57	9	0.2	39	0.8	310	432	70	20	0.04	0.10	1.4	2	250
45	3	0.0	98	2.6	405	225	85	26	0.09	0.05	1.1	0	251
150	10	0.3	57	1.1	191	292	161	48	0.11	0.12	2.6	1	252
80	5	0.2	30	0.6	101	155	85	25	0.06	0.06	1.4	1	253
147	1	0.0	50	2.3	179	144	51	15	0.02	0.03	2.3	2	254
43	0	0.0	5	0.9	314	98	116	35	0.04	0.10	10.0	1	255
53	0	0.0	6	1.1	391	122	145	43	0.05	0.12	12.5	1	256
58	0	0.0	73	0.3	375	36	244	73	0.20	0.07	7.5	3	257
48	0	0.0	61	0.2	313	30	204	61	0.17	0.06	6.2	2	258
49	0	0.0	18	0.8	484	40	58	17	0.43	0.05	10.1	1	259
15	0	0.0	11	1.2	176	301	66	20	0.03	0.10	10.5	0	260
26	0	0.0	9	1.3	201	287	48	14	0.03	0.06	11.3	0	261
36	0	0.0	12	0.8	201	320	16	5	0.01	0.04	4.9	0	262
27	19	0.0	35	2.1	365	824	199	55	0.06	0.14	13.7	5	263
0	21	3.7	10	0.2	159	0	73	7	0.02	0.02	0.1	8	264
0	16	2.1	4	0.1	124	0	48	4	0.02	0.01	0.1	4	265
0	21	2.8	4	0.4	144	28	0	0	0.00	0.05	0.3	1	266
0	29	0.2	17	0.9	295	7	2	0	0.05	0.04	0.2	2	267
0	19	0.7	3	0.2	33	33	10	1	0.01	0.01	Tr	1	268
0	51	3.1	10	0.9	156	8	28	3	0.03	0.07	0.5	4	269
0	28	2.9	7	0.3	183	5	71	7	0.03	0.06	0.5	3	270
0	4	0.8	5	0.2	104	Tr	914	91	0.01	0.01	0.2	4	271
0	55	4.1	23	0.8	361	10	3,173	317	0.05	0.06	1.0	8	272
0	30	3.9	29	0.7	403	10	4,126	412	0.04	0.05	0.8	12	273
0	22	3.2	16	1.6	482	4	2,534	253	Tr	0.05	1.0	1	274
0	36	1.5	18	1.0	286	8	3,303	331	0.02	0.04	0.7	137	275
0	13	4.4	5	0.0	148	0	0	0	0.01	0.01	0.3	5	276
0	29	9.9	11	0.0	333	0	0	0	0.02	0.03	0.6	10	277

Table 9. Nutritive Value of the Edible Part of Food

Food No.	Food Description	Measure of edible portion	Weight (g)	Water (%)	Calories (kcal)	Protein (g)	Total fat (g)	Fatty acids Saturated (g)	Fatty acids Mono- unsaturated (g)	Fatty acids Poly- unsaturated (g)
	Fruits and Fruit Juices (continued)									
	Avocados, raw, without skin and seed									
278	California (about ⅕ whole)	1 oz	28	73	50	1	5	0.7	3.2	0.6
279	Florida (about ⅒ whole)	1 oz	28	80	32	Tr	3	0.5	1.4	0.4
	Bananas, raw									
280	Whole, medium (7" to 7⅞" long)	1 banana	118	74	109	1	1	0.2	Tr	0.1
281	Sliced	1 cup	150	74	138	2	1	0.3	0.1	0.1
282	Blackberries, raw	1 cup	144	86	75	1	1	Tr	0.1	0.3
	Blueberries									
283	Raw	1 cup	145	85	81	1	1	Tr	0.1	0.2
284	Frozen, sweetened, thawed	1 cup	230	77	186	1	Tr	Tr	Tr	0.1
	Cantaloupe. See Melons.									
	Carambola (starfruit), raw									
285	Whole (3⅝" long)	1 fruit	91	91	30	Tr	Tr	Tr	Tr	0.2
286	Sliced	1 cup	108	91	36	1	Tr	Tr	Tr	0.2
	Cherries									
287	Sour, red, pitted, canned, water pack	1 cup	244	90	88	2	Tr	0.1	0.1	0.1
288	Sweet, raw, without pits and stems	10 cherries	68	81	49	1	1	0.1	0.2	0.2
289	Cherry pie filling, canned	⅛ of 21-oz can	74	71	85	Tr	Tr	Tr	Tr	Tr
290	Cranberries, dried, sweetened	¼ cup	28	12	92	Tr	Tr	Tr	Tr	0.1
291	Cranberry sauce, sweetened, canned (about 8 slices per can)	1 slice	57	61	86	Tr	Tr	Tr	Tr	Tr
	Dates, without pits									
292	Whole	5 dates	42	23	116	1	Tr	0.1	0.1	Tr
293	Chopped	1 cup	178	23	490	4	1	0.3	0.3	0.1
294	Figs, dried	2 figs	38	28	97	1	Tr	0.1	0.1	0.2
	Fruit cocktail, canned, fruit and liquid									
295	Heavy syrup pack	1 cup	248	80	181	1	Tr	Tr	Tr	0.1
296	Juice pack	1 cup	237	87	109	1	Tr	Tr	Tr	Tr
	Grapefruit									
	Raw, without peel, membrane and seeds (3¾" dia)									
297	Pink or red	½ grapefruit	123	91	37	1	Tr	Tr	Tr	Tr
298	White	½ grapefruit	118	90	39	1	Tr	Tr	Tr	Tr
299	Canned, sections with light syrup	1 cup	254	84	152	1	Tr	Tr	Tr	0.1
	Grapefruit juice									
	Raw									
300	Pink	1 cup	247	90	96	1	Tr	Tr	Tr	0.1
301	White	1 cup	247	90	96	1	Tr	Tr	Tr	0.1
	Canned									
302	Unsweetened	1 cup	247	90	94	1	Tr	Tr	Tr	0.1
303	Sweetened	1 cup	250	87	115	1	Tr	Tr	Tr	0.1
	Frozen concentrate, unsweetened									
304	Undiluted	6-fl-oz can	207	62	302	4	1	0.1	0.1	0.2
305	Diluted with 3 parts water by volume	1 cup	247	89	101	1	Tr	Tr	Tr	0.1
306	Grapes, seedless, raw	10 grapes	50	81	36	Tr	Tr	0.1	Tr	0.1
307		1 cup	160	81	114	1	1	0.3	Tr	0.3

Choles-terol (mg)	Carbo-hydrate (g)	Total dietary fiber (g)	Calcium (mg)	Iron (mg)	Potas-sium (mg)	Sodium (mg)	Vitamin A (IU)	Vitamin A (RE)	Thiamin (mg)	Ribo-flavin (mg)	Niacin (mg)	Ascor-bic acid (mg)	Food No.
0	2	1.4	3	0.3	180	3	174	17	0.03	0.03	0.5	2	278
0	3	1.5	3	0.2	138	1	174	17	0.03	0.03	0.5	2	279
0	28	2.8	7	0.4	467	1	96	9	0.05	0.12	0.6	11	280
0	35	3.6	9	0.5	594	2	122	12	0.07	0.15	0.8	14	281
0	18	7.6	46	0.8	282	0	238	23	0.04	0.06	0.6	30	282
0	20	3.9	9	0.2	129	9	145	15	0.07	0.07	0.5	19	283
0	50	4.8	14	0.9	138	2	101	9	0.05	0.12	0.6	2	284
0	7	2.5	4	0.2	148	2	449	45	0.03	0.02	0.4	19	285
0	8	2.9	4	0.3	176	2	532	53	0.03	0.03	0.4	23	286
0	22	2.7	27	3.3	239	17	1,840	183	0.04	0.10	0.4	5	287
0	11	1.6	10	0.3	152	0	146	14	0.03	0.04	0.3	5	288
0	21	0.4	8	0.2	78	13	152	16	0.02	0.01	0.1	3	289
0	24	2.5	5	0.1	24	1	0	0	0.01	0.03	Tr	Tr	290
0	22	0.6	2	0.1	15	17	11	1	0.01	0.01	0.1	1	291
0	31	3.2	13	0.5	274	1	21	2	0.04	0.04	0.9	0	292
0	131	13.4	57	2.0	1,161	5	89	9	0.16	0.18	3.9	0	293
0	25	4.6	55	0.8	271	4	51	5	0.03	0.03	0.3	Tr	294
0	47	2.5	15	0.7	218	15	508	50	0.04	0.05	0.9	5	295
0	28	2.4	19	0.5	225	9	723	73	0.03	0.04	1.0	6	296
0	9	1.4	14	0.1	159	0	319	32	0.04	0.02	0.2	47	297
0	10	1.3	14	0.1	175	0	12	1	0.04	0.02	0.3	39	298
0	39	1.0	36	1.0	328	5	0	0	0.10	0.05	0.6	54	299
0	23	0.2	22	0.5	400	2	1,087	109	0.10	0.05	0.5	94	300
0	23	0.2	22	0.5	400	2	25	2	0.10	0.05	0.5	94	301
0	22	0.2	17	0.5	378	2	17	2	0.10	0.05	0.6	72	302
0	28	0.3	20	0.9	405	5	0	0	0.10	0.06	0.8	67	303
0	72	0.8	56	1.0	1,002	6	64	6	0.30	0.16	1.6	248	304
0	24	0.2	20	0.3	336	2	22	2	0.10	0.05	0.5	83	305
0	9	0.5	6	0.1	93	1	37	4	0.05	0.03	0.2	5	306
0	28	1.6	18	0.4	296	3	117	11	0.15	0.09	0.5	17	307

Table 9. Nutritive Value of the Edible Part of Food

Food No.	Food Description	Measure of edible portion	Weight (g)	Water (%)	Calories (kcal)	Protein (g)	Total fat (g)	Fatty acids Saturated (g)	Mono- unsaturated (g)	Poly- unsaturated (g)
	Fruits and Fruit Juices (continued)									
	Grape juice									
308	Canned or bottled	1 cup	253	84	154	1	Tr	0.1	Tr	0.1
	Frozen concentrate, sweetened, with added vitamin C									
309	Undiluted	6-fl-oz can	216	54	387	1	1	0.2	Tr	0.2
310	Diluted with 3 parts water by volume	1 cup	250	87	128	Tr	Tr	0.1	Tr	0.1
311	Kiwi fruit, raw, without skin (about 5 per lb with skin)	1 medium	76	83	46	1	Tr	Tr	Tr	0.2
312	Lemons, raw, without peel (2⅛" dia with peel)	1 lemon	58	89	17	1	Tr	Tr	Tr	0.1
	Lemon juice									
313	Raw (from 2⅛"-dia lemon)	juice of 1 lemon	47	91	12	Tr	0	0.0	0.0	0.0
314	Canned or bottled, unsweetened	1 cup	244	92	51	1	1	0.1	Tr	0.2
315		1 tbsp	15	92	3	Tr	Tr	Tr	Tr	Tr
	Lime juice									
316	Raw (from 2"-dia lime)	juice of 1 lime	38	90	10	Tr	Tr	Tr	Tr	Tr
317	Canned, unsweetened	1 cup	246	93	52	1	1	0.1	0.1	0.2
318		1 tbsp	15	93	3	Tr	Tr	Tr	Tr	Tr
	Mangos, raw, without skin and seed (about 1½ per lb with skin and seed)									
319	Whole	1 mango	207	82	135	1	1	0.1	0.2	0.1
320	Sliced	1 cup	165	82	107	1	Tr	0.1	0.2	0.1
	Melons, raw, without rind and cavity contents									
	Cantaloupe (5" dia)									
321	Wedge	⅛ melon	69	90	24	1	Tr	Tr	Tr	0.1
322	Cubes	1 cup	160	90	56	1	Tr	0.1	Tr	0.2
	Honeydew (6"-7" dia)									
323	Wedge	⅛ melon	160	90	56	1	Tr	Tr	Tr	0.1
324	Diced (about 20 pieces per cup)	1 cup	170	90	60	1	Tr	Tr	Tr	0.1
325	Mixed fruit, frozen, sweetened, thawed (peach, cherry, raspberry, grape and boysenberry)	1 cup	250	74	245	4	Tr	0.1	0.1	0.2
326	Nectarines, raw (2½" dia)	1 nectarine	136	86	67	1	1	0.1	0.2	0.3
	Oranges, raw									
327	Whole, without peel and seeds (2⅝" dia)	1 orange	131	87	62	1	Tr	Tr	Tr	Tr
328	Sections without membranes	1 cup	180	87	85	2	Tr	Tr	Tr	Tr
	Orange juice									
329	Raw, all varieties	1 cup	248	88	112	2	Tr	0.1	0.1	0.1
330		juice from 1 orange	86	88	39	1	Tr	Tr	Tr	Tr
331	Canned, unsweetened	1 cup	249	89	105	1	Tr	Tr	0.1	0.1
332	Chilled (refrigerator case)	1 cup	249	88	110	2	1	0.1	0.1	0.2
	Frozen concentrate									
333	Undiluted	6-fl-oz can	213	58	339	5	Tr	0.1	0.1	0.1
334	Diluted with 3 parts water by volume	1 cup	249	88	112	2	Tr	Tr	Tr	Tr
	Papayas, raw									
335	½" cubes	1 cup	140	89	55	1	Tr	0.1	0.1	Tr
336	Whole (5⅛" long x 3" dia)	1 papaya	304	89	119	2	Tr	0.1	0.1	0.1

*Sodium benzoate and sodium bisulfite added as preservatives.

Choles- terol (mg)	Carbo- hydrate (g)	Total dietary fiber (g)	Calcium (mg)	Iron (mg)	Potas- sium (mg)	Sodium (mg)	Vitamin A (IU)	Vitamin A (RE)	Thiamin (mg)	Ribo- flavin (mg)	Niacin (mg)	Ascor- bic acid (mg)	Food No.
0	38	0.3	23	0.6	334	8	20	3	0.07	0.09	0.7	Tr	308
0	96	0.6	28	0.8	160	15	58	6	0.11	0.20	0.9	179	309
0	32	0.3	10	0.3	53	5	20	3	0.04	0.07	0.3	60	310
0	11	2.6	20	0.3	252	4	133	14	0.02	0.04	0.4	74	311
0	5	1.6	15	0.3	80	1	17	2	0.02	0.01	0.1	31	312
0	4	0.2	3	Tr	58	Tr	9	1	0.01	Tr	Tr	22	313
0	16	1.0	27	0.3	249	51*	37	5	0.10	0.02	0.5	61	314
0	1	0.1	2	Tr	16	3*	2	Tr	0.01	Tr	Tr	4	315
0	3	0.2	3	Tr	41	Tr	4	Tr	0.01	Tr	Tr	11	316
0	16	1.0	30	0.6	185	39*	39	5	0.08	0.01	0.4	16	317
0	1	0.1	2	Tr	11	2*	2	Tr	Tr	Tr	Tr	1	318
0	35	3.7	21	0.3	323	4	8,061	805	0.12	0.12	1.2	57	319
0	28	3.0	17	0.2	257	3	6,425	642	0.10	0.09	1.0	46	320
0	6	0.6	8	0.1	213	6	2,225	222	0.02	0.01	0.4	29	321
0	13	1.3	18	0.3	494	14	5,158	515	0.06	0.03	0.9	68	322
0	15	1.0	10	0.1	434	16	64	6	0.12	0.03	1.0	40	323
0	16	1.0	10	0.1	461	17	68	7	0.13	0.03	1.0	42	324
0	61	4.8	18	0.7	328	8	805	80	0.04	0.09	1.0	188	325
0	16	2.2	7	0.2	288	0	1,001	101	0.02	0.06	1.3	7	326
0	15	3.1	52	0.1	237	0	269	28	0.11	0.05	0.4	70	327
0	21	4.3	72	0.2	326	0	369	38	0.16	0.07	0.5	96	328
0	26	0.5	27	0.5	496	2	496	50	0.22	0.07	1.0	124	329
0	9	0.2	9	0.2	172	1	172	17	0.08	0.03	0.3	43	330
0	25	0.5	20	1.1	436	5	436	45	0.15	0.07	0.8	86	331
0	25	0.5	25	0.4	473	2	194	20	0.28	0.05	0.7	82	332
0	81	1.7	68	0.7	1,436	6	588	60	0.60	0.14	1.5	294	333
0	27	0.5	22	0.2	473	2	194	20	0.20	0.04	0.5	97	334
0	14	2.5	34	0.1	360	4	398	39	0.04	0.04	0.5	87	335
0	30	5.5	73	0.3	781	9	863	85	0.08	0.10	1.0	188	336

Table 9. Nutritive Value of the Edible Part of Food

Food No.	Food Description	Measure of edible portion	Weight (g)	Water (%)	Calories (kcal)	Protein (g)	Total fat (g)	Saturated (g)	Mono-unsaturated (g)	Poly-unsaturated (g)
	Fruits and Fruit Juices (continued)									
	Peaches									
	Raw									
337	Whole, 2½" dia, pitted (about 4 per lb)	1 peach	98	88	42	1	Tr	Tr	Tr	Tr
338	Sliced	1 cup	170	88	73	1	Tr	Tr	0.1	0.1
	Canned, fruit and liquid									
339	Heavy syrup pack	1 cup	262	79	194	1	Tr	Tr	0.1	0.1
340		1 half	98	79	73	Tr	Tr	Tr	Tr	Tr
341	Juice pack	1 cup	248	87	109	2	Tr	Tr	Tr	Tr
342		1 half	98	87	43	1	Tr	Tr	Tr	Tr
343	Dried, sulfured	3 halves	39	32	93	1	Tr	Tr	0.1	0.1
344	Frozen, sliced, sweetened, with added ascorbic acid, thawed	1 cup	250	75	235	2	Tr	Tr	0.1	0.2
	Pears									
345	Raw, with skin, cored, 2½" dia	1 pear	166	84	98	1	1	Tr	0.1	0.2
	Canned, fruit and liquid									
346	Heavy syrup pack	1 cup	266	80	197	1	Tr	Tr	0.1	0.1
347		1 half	76	80	56	Tr	Tr	Tr	Tr	Tr
348	Juice pack	1 cup	248	86	124	1	Tr	Tr	Tr	Tr
349		1 half	76	86	38	Tr	Tr	Tr	Tr	Tr
	Pineapple									
350	Raw, diced	1 cup	155	87	76	1	1	Tr	0.1	0.2
	Canned, fruit and liquid									
	Heavy syrup pack									
351	Crushed, sliced, or chunks	1 cup	254	79	198	1	Tr	Tr	Tr	0.1
352	Slices (3" dia)	1 slice	49	79	38	Tr	Tr	Tr	Tr	Tr
	Juice pack									
353	Crushed, sliced, or chunks	1 cup	249	84	149	1	Tr	Tr	Tr	0.1
354	Slice (3" dia)	1 slice	47	84	28	Tr	Tr	Tr	Tr	Tr
355	Pineapple juice, unsweetened, canned	1 cup	250	86	140	1	Tr	Tr	Tr	0.1
	Plantain, without peel									
356	Raw	1 medium	179	65	218	2	1	0.3	0.1	0.1
357	Cooked, slices	1 cup	154	67	179	1	Tr	0.1	Tr	0.1
	Plums									
358	Raw (2⅛" dia)	1 plum	66	85	36	1	Tr	Tr	0.3	0.1
	Canned, purple, fruit and liquid									
359	Heavy syrup pack	1 cup	258	76	230	1	Tr	Tr	0.2	0.1
360		1 plum	46	76	41	Tr	Tr	Tr	Tr	Tr
361	Juice pack	1 cup	252	84	146	1	Tr	Tr	Tr	Tr
362		1 plum	46	84	27	Tr	Tr	Tr	Tr	Tr
	Prunes, dried, pitted									
363	Uncooked	5 prunes	42	32	100	1	Tr	Tr	0.1	Tr
364	Stewed, unsweetened, fruit and liquid	1 cup	248	70	265	3	1	Tr	0.4	0.1
365	Prune juice, canned or bottled	1 cup	256	81	182	2	Tr	Tr	0.1	Tr
	Raisins, seedless									
366	Cup, not packed	1 cup	145	15	435	5	1	0.2	Tr	0.2
367	Packet, ½ oz (1½ tbsp)	1 packet	14	15	42	Tr	Tr	Tr	Tr	Tr
	Raspberries									
368	Raw	1 cup	123	87	60	1	1	Tr	0.1	0.4
369	Frozen, sweetened, thawed	1 cup	250	73	258	2	Tr	Tr	Tr	0.2
370	Rhubarb, frozen, cooked, with sugar	1 cup	240	68	278	1	Tr	Tr	Tr	0.1

Choles-terol (mg)	Carbo-hydrate (g)	Total dietary fiber (g)	Calcium (mg)	Iron (mg)	Potas-sium (mg)	Sodium (mg)	Vitamin A		Thiamin (mg)	Ribo-flavin (mg)	Niacin (mg)	Ascor-bic acid (mg)	Food No.
							(IU)	(RE)					
0	11	2.0	5	0.1	193	0	524	53	0.02	0.04	1.0	6	337
0	19	3.4	9	0.2	335	0	910	92	0.03	0.07	1.7	11	338
0	52	3.4	8	0.7	241	16	870	86	0.03	0.06	1.6	7	339
0	20	1.3	3	0.3	90	6	325	32	0.01	0.02	0.6	3	340
0	29	3.2	15	0.7	317	10	945	94	0.02	0.04	1.4	9	341
0	11	1.3	6	0.3	125	4	373	37	0.01	0.02	0.6	4	342
0	24	3.2	11	1.6	388	3	844	84	Tr	0.08	1.7	2	343
0	60	4.5	8	0.9	325	15	710	70	0.03	0.09	1.6	236	344
0	25	4.0	18	0.4	208	0	33	3	0.03	0.07	0.2	7	345
0	51	4.3	13	0.6	173	13	0	0	0.03	0.06	0.6	3	346
0	15	1.2	4	0.2	49	4	0	0	0.01	0.02	0.2	1	347
0	32	4.0	22	0.7	238	10	15	2	0.03	0.03	0.5	4	348
0	10	1.2	7	0.2	73	3	5	1	0.01	0.01	0.2	1	349
0	19	1.9	11	0.6	175	2	36	3	0.14	0.06	0.7	24	350
0	51	2.0	36	1.0	264	3	36	3	0.23	0.06	0.7	19	351
0	10	0.4	7	0.2	51	Tr	7	Tr	0.04	0.01	0.1	4	352
0	39	2.0	35	0.7	304	2	95	10	0.24	0.05	0.7	24	353
0	7	0.4	7	0.1	57	Tr	18	2	0.04	0.01	0.1	4	354
0	34	0.5	43	0.7	335	3	13	0	0.14	0.06	0.6	27	355
0	57	4.1	5	1.1	893	7	2,017	202	0.09	0.10	1.2	33	356
0	48	3.5	3	0.9	716	8	1,400	140	0.07	0.08	1.2	17	357
0	9	1.0	3	0.1	114	0	213	21	0.03	0.06	0.3	6	358
0	60	2.6	23	2.2	235	49	668	67	0.04	0.10	0.8	1	359
0	11	0.5	4	0.4	42	9	119	12	0.01	0.02	0.1	Tr	360
0	38	2.5	25	0.9	388	3	2,543	255	0.06	0.15	1.2	7	361
0	7	0.5	5	0.2	71	Tr	464	46	0.01	0.03	0.2	1	362
0	26	3.0	21	1.0	313	2	835	84	0.03	0.07	0.8	1	363
0	70	16.4	57	2.8	828	5	759	77	0.06	0.25	1.8	7	364
0	45	2.6	31	3.0	707	10	8	0	0.04	0.18	2.0	10	365
0	115	5.8	71	3.0	1,089	17	12	1	0.23	0.13	1.2	5	366
0	11	0.6	7	0.3	105	2	1	Tr	0.02	0.01	0.1	Tr	367
0	14	8.4	27	0.7	187	0	160	16	0.04	0.11	1.1	31	368
0	65	11.0	38	1.6	285	3	150	15	0.05	0.11	0.6	41	369
0	75	4.8	348	0.5	230	2	166	17	0.04	0.06	0.5	8	370

Table 9. Nutritive Value of the Edible Part of Food

Food No.	Food Description	Measure of edible portion	Weight (g)	Water (%)	Calories (kcal)	Protein (g)	Total fat (g)	Fatty acids		
								Saturated (g)	Mono-unsaturated (g)	Poly-unsaturated (g)

Fruits and Fruit Juices (continued)

Strawberries
  Raw, capped

371	Large (1⅛" dia)	1 strawberry	18	92	5	Tr	Tr	Tr	Tr	Tr
372	Medium (1¼" dia)	1 strawberry	12	92	4	Tr	Tr	Tr	Tr	Tr
373	Sliced	1 cup	166	92	50	1	1	Tr	0.1	0.3
374	Frozen, sweetened, sliced, thawed	1 cup	255	73	245	1	Tr	Tr	Tr	0.2

Tangerines

375	Raw, without peel and seeds (2⅜" dia)	1 tangerine	84	88	37	1	Tr	Tr	Tr	Tr
376	Canned (mandarin oranges), light syrup, fruit and liquid	1 cup	252	83	154	1	Tr	Tr	Tr	0.1
377	Tangerine juice, canned, sweetened	1 cup	249	87	125	1	Tr	Tr	Tr	0.1

Watermelon, raw (15" long x 7½" dia)

378	Wedge (about 1/16 of melon)	1 wedge	286	92	92	2	1	0.1	0.3	0.4
379	Diced	1 cup	152	92	49	1	1	0.1	0.2	0.2

Grain Products

Bagels, enriched

380	Plain	3½" bagel	71	33	195	7	1	0.2	0.1	0.5
381		4" bagel	89	33	245	9	1	0.2	0.1	0.6
382	Cinnamon raisin	3½" bagel	71	32	195	7	1	0.2	0.1	0.5
383		4" bagel	89	32	244	9	2	0.2	0.2	0.6
384	Egg	3½" bagel	71	33	197	8	1	0.3	0.3	0.5
385		4" bagel	89	33	247	9	2	0.4	0.4	0.6
386	Banana bread, prepared from recipe, with margarine	1 slice	60	29	196	3	6	1.3	2.7	1.9

Barley, pearled

387	Uncooked	1 cup	200	10	704	20	2	0.5	0.3	1.1
388	Cooked	1 cup	157	69	193	4	1	0.1	0.1	0.3

Biscuits, plain or buttermilk, enriched

389	Prepared from recipe, with 2% milk	2½" biscuit	60	29	212	4	10	2.6	4.2	2.5
390		4" biscuit	101	29	358	7	16	4.4	7.0	4.2

Refrigerated dough, baked

391	Regular	2½" biscuit	27	28	93	2	4	1.0	2.2	0.5
392	Lower fat	2¼" biscuit	21	28	63	2	1	0.3	0.6	0.2

Breads, enriched

393	Cracked wheat	1 slice	25	36	65	2	1	0.2	0.5	0.2
394	Egg bread (challah)	½" slice	40	35	115	4	2	0.6	0.9	0.4
395	French or vienna (includes sourdough)	½" slice	25	34	69	2	1	0.2	0.3	0.2
396	Indian fry (navajo) bread	5" bread	90	27	296	6	9	2.1	3.6	2.3
397		10½" bread	160	27	526	11	15	3.7	6.4	4.1
398	Italian	1 slice	20	36	54	2	1	0.2	0.2	0.3

Mixed grain

399	Untoasted	1 slice	26	38	65	3	1	0.2	0.4	0.2
400	Toasted	1 slice	24	32	65	3	1	0.2	0.4	0.2

Oatmeal

401	Untoasted	1 slice	27	37	73	2	1	0.2	0.4	0.5
402	Toasted	1 slice	25	31	73	2	1	0.2	0.4	0.5
403	Pita	4" pita	28	32	77	3	Tr	Tr	Tr	0.1
404		6½" pita	60	32	165	5	1	0.1	0.1	0.3

Choles-terol (mg)	Carbo-hydrate (g)	Total dietary fiber (g)	Calcium (mg)	Iron (mg)	Potas-sium (mg)	Sodium (mg)	Vitamin A (IU)	Vitamin A (RE)	Thiamin (mg)	Ribo-flavin (mg)	Niacin (mg)	Ascor-bic acid (mg)	Food No.
0	1	0.4	3	0.1	30	Tr	5	1	Tr	0.01	Tr	10	371
0	1	0.3	2	Tr	20	Tr	3	Tr	Tr	0.01	Tr	7	372
0	12	3.8	23	0.6	276	2	45	5	0.03	0.11	0.4	94	373
0	66	4.8	28	1.5	250	8	61	5	0.04	0.13	1.0	106	374
0	9	1.9	12	0.1	132	1	773	77	0.09	0.02	0.1	26	375
0	41	1.8	18	0.9	197	15	2,117	212	0.13	0.11	1.1	50	376
0	30	0.5	45	0.5	443	2	1,046	105	0.15	0.05	0.2	55	377
0	21	1.4	23	0.5	332	6	1,047	106	0.23	0.06	0.6	27	378
0	11	0.8	12	0.3	176	3	556	56	0.12	0.03	0.3	15	379
0	38	1.6	53	2.5	72	379	0	0	0.38	0.22	3.2	0	380
0	48	2.0	66	3.2	90	475	0	0	0.48	0.28	4.1	0	381
0	39	1.6	13	2.7	105	229	52	0	0.27	0.20	2.2	Tr	382
0	49	2.0	17	3.4	132	287	65	0	0.34	0.25	2.7	1	383
17	38	1.6	9	2.8	48	359	77	23	0.38	0.17	2.4	Tr	384
21	47	2.0	12	3.5	61	449	97	29	0.48	0.21	3.1	1	385
26	33	0.7	13	0.8	80	181	278	72	0.10	0.12	0.9	1	386
0	155	31.2	58	5.0	560	18	44	4	0.38	0.23	9.2	0	387
0	44	6.0	17	2.1	146	5	11	2	0.13	0.10	3.2	0	388
2	27	0.9	141	1.7	73	348	49	14	0.21	0.19	1.8	Tr	389
3	45	1.5	237	2.9	122	586	83	23	0.36	0.31	3.0	Tr	390
0	13	0.4	5	0.7	42	325	0	0	0.09	0.06	0.8	0	391
0	12	0.4	4	0.6	39	305	0	0	0.09	0.05	0.7	0	392
0	12	1.4	11	0.7	44	135	0	0	0.09	0.06	0.9	0	393
20	19	0.9	37	1.2	46	197	30	9	0.18	0.17	1.9	0	394
0	13	0.8	19	0.6	28	152	0	0	0.13	0.08	1.2	0	395
0	48	1.6	210	3.2	67	626	0	0	0.39	0.27	3.3	0	396
0	85	2.9	373	5.8	118	1,112	0	0	0.69	0.49	5.8	0	397
0	10	0.5	16	0.6	22	117	0	0	0.09	0.06	0.9	0	398
0	12	1.7	24	0.9	53	127	0	0	0.11	0.09	1.1	Tr	399
0	12	1.6	24	0.9	53	127	0	0	0.08	0.08	1.0	Tr	400
0	13	1.1	18	0.7	38	162	4	1	0.11	0.06	0.8	0	401
0	13	1.1	18	0.7	39	163	4	1	0.09	0.06	0.8	Tr	402
0	16	0.6	24	0.7	34	150	0	0	0.17	0.09	1.3	0	403
0	33	1.3	52	1.6	72	322	0	0	0.36	0.20	2.8	0	404

Table 9. Nutritive Value of the Edible Part of Food

Food No.	Food Description	Measure of edible portion	Weight (g)	Water (%)	Calories (kcal)	Protein (g)	Total fat (g)	Fatty acids Saturated (g)	Mono-unsaturated (g)	Poly-unsaturated (g)
	Grain Products (continued)									
	Breads, enriched (continued)									
	Pumpernickel									
405	Untoasted	1 slice	32	38	80	3	1	0.1	0.3	0.4
406	Toasted	1 slice	29	32	80	3	1	0.1	0.3	0.4
	Raisin									
407	Untoasted	1 slice	26	34	71	2	1	0.3	0.6	0.2
408	Toasted	1 slice	24	28	71	2	1	0.3	0.6	0.2
	Rye									
409	Untoasted	1 slice	32	37	83	3	1	0.2	0.4	0.3
410	Toasted	1 slice	24	31	68	2	1	0.2	0.3	0.2
411	Rye, reduced calorie	1 slice	23	46	47	2	1	0.1	0.2	0.2
	Wheat									
412	Untoasted	1 slice	25	37	65	2	1	0.2	0.4	0.2
413	Toasted	1 slice	23	32	65	2	1	0.2	0.4	0.2
414	Wheat, reduced calorie	1 slice	23	43	46	2	1	0.1	0.1	0.2
	White									
415	Untoasted	1 slice	25	37	67	2	1	0.1	0.2	0.5
416	Toasted	1 slice	22	30	64	2	1	0.1	0.2	0.5
417	Soft crumbs	1 cup	45	37	120	4	2	0.2	0.3	0.9
418	White, reduced calorie	1 slice	23	43	48	2	1	0.1	0.2	0.1
	Bread, whole wheat									
419	Untoasted	1 slice	28	38	69	3	1	0.3	0.5	0.3
420	Toasted	1 slice	25	30	69	3	1	0.3	0.5	0.3
	Bread crumbs, dry, grated									
421	Plain, enriched	1 cup	108	6	427	14	6	1.3	2.6	1.2
422		1 oz	28	6	112	4	2	0.3	0.7	0.3
423	Seasoned, unenriched	1 cup	120	6	440	17	3	0.9	1.2	0.8
	Bread crumbs, soft. See White bread.									
424	Bread stuffing, prepared from dry mix	½ cup	100	65	178	3	9	1.7	3.8	2.6
425	Breakfast bar, cereal crust with fruit filling, fat free	1 bar	37	14	121	2	Tr	Tr	Tr	0.1
	Breakfast Cereals									
	Hot type, cooked									
	Corn (hominy) grits									
	Regular or quick, enriched									
426	White	1 cup	242	85	145	3	Tr	0.1	0.1	0.2
427	Yellow	1 cup	242	85	145	3	Tr	0.1	0.1	0.2
428	Instant, plain	1 packet	137	82	89	2	Tr	Tr	Tr	0.1
	CREAM OF WHEAT									
429	Regular	1 cup	251	87	133	4	1	0.1	0.1	0.3
430	Quick	1 cup	239	87	129	4	Tr	0.1	0.1	0.3
431	Mix'n Eat, plain	1 packet	142	82	102	3	Tr	Tr	Tr	0.2
432	MALT O MEAL	1 cup	240	88	122	4	Tr	0.1	0.1	Tr
	Oatmeal									
433	Regular, quick or instant, plain, nonfortified	1 cup	234	85	145	6	2	0.4	0.7	0.9
434	Instant, fortified, plain	1 packet	177	86	104	4	2	0.3	0.6	0.7
	QUAKER instant									
435	Apples and cinnamon	1 packet	149	79	125	3	1	0.3	0.5	0.6
436	Maple and brown sugar	1 packet	155	75	153	4	2	0.4	0.6	0.7
437	WHEATENA	1 cup	243	85	136	5	1	0.2	0.2	0.6
	Ready to eat									
438	ALL BRAN	½ cup	30	3	79	4	1	0.2	0.2	0.5
439	APPLE CINNAMON CHEERIOS	¾ cup	30	3	118	2	2	0.3	0.6	0.2
440	APPLE JACKS	1 cup	30	3	116	1	Tr	0.1	0.1	0.2

Choles-terol (mg)	Carbo-hydrate (g)	Total dietary fiber (g)	Calcium (mg)	Iron (mg)	Potas-sium (mg)	Sodium (mg)	Vitamin A (IU)	Vitamin A (RE)	Thiamin (mg)	Ribo-flavin (mg)	Niacin (mg)	Ascor-bic acid (mg)	Food No.
0	15	2.1	22	0.9	67	215	0	0	0.10	0.10	1.0	0	405
0	15	2.1	21	0.9	66	214	0	0	0.08	0.09	0.9	0	406
0	14	1.1	17	0.8	59	101	0	0	0.09	0.10	0.9	Tr	407
0	14	1.1	17	0.8	59	102	Tr	0	0.07	0.09	0.8	Tr	408
0	15	1.9	23	0.9	53	211	2	Tr	0.14	0.11	1.2	Tr	409
0	13	1.5	19	0.7	44	174	1	0	0.09	0.08	0.9	Tr	410
0	9	2.8	17	0.7	23	93	1	0	0.08	0.06	0.6	Tr	411
0	12	1.1	26	0.8	50	133	0	0	0.10	0.07	1.0	0	412
0	12	1.2	26	0.8	50	132	0	0	0.08	0.06	0.9	0	413
0	10	2.8	18	0.7	28	118	0	0	0.10	0.07	0.9	Tr	414
Tr	12	0.6	27	0.8	30	135	0	0	0.12	0.09	1.0	0	415
Tr	12	0.6	26	0.7	29	130	0	0	0.09	0.07	0.9	0	416
Tr	22	1.0	49	1.4	54	242	0	0	0.21	0.15	1.8	0	417
0	10	2.2	22	0.7	17	104	1	Tr	0.09	0.07	0.8	Tr	418
0	13	1.9	20	0.9	71	148	0	0	0.10	0.06	1.1	0	419
0	13	1.9	20	0.9	71	148	0	0	0.08	0.05	1.0	0	420
0	78	2.6	245	6.6	239	931	1	0	0.83	0.47	7.4	0	421
0	21	0.7	64	1.7	63	244	Tr	0	0.22	0.12	1.9	0	422
1	84	5.0	119	3.8	324	3,180	16	4	0.19	0.20	3.3	Tr	423
0	22	2.9	32	1.1	74	543	313	81	0.14	0.11	1.5	0	424
Tr	28	0.8	49	4.5	92	203	1,249	125	1.01	0.42	5.0	1	425
0	31	0.5	0	1.5	53	0	0	0	0.24	0.15	2.0	0	426
0	31	0.5	0	1.5	53	0	145	15	0.24	0.15	2.0	0	427
0	21	1.2	8	8.2	38	289	0	0	0.15	0.08	1.4	0	428
0	28	1.8	50	10.3	43	3	0	0	0.25	0.00	1.5	0	429
0	27	1.2	50	10.3	45	139	0	0	0.24	0.00	1.4	0	430
0	21	0.4	20	8.1	38	241	1,252	376	0.43	0.28	5.0	0	431
0	26	1.0	5	9.6	31	2	0	0	0.48	0.24	5.8	0	432
0	25	4.0	19	1.6	131	2	37	5	0.26	0.05	0.3	0	433
0	18	3.0	163	6.3	99	285	1,510	453	0.53	0.28	5.5	0	434
0	26	2.5	104	3.9	106	121	1,019	305	0.30	0.35	4.1	Tr	435
0	31	2.6	105	3.9	112	234	1,008	302	0.30	0.34	4.0	0	436
0	29	6.6	10	1.4	187	5	0	0	0.02	0.05	1.3	0	437
0	23	9.7	106	4.5	342	61	750	225	0.39	0.42	5.0	15	438
0	25	1.6	35	4.5	60	150	750	225	0.38	0.43	5.0	15	439
0	27	0.6	3	4.5	32	134	750	225	0.39	0.42	5.0	15	440

Table 9. Nutritive Value of the Edible Part of Food

Food No.	Food Description	Measure of edible portion	Weight (g)	Water (%)	Calories (kcal)	Protein (g)	Total fat (g)	Fatty acids Saturated (g)	Mono-unsaturated (g)	Poly-unsaturated (g)
	Grain Products (continued)									
	Breakfast Cereals (continued)									
	Ready to eat (continued)									
441	BASIC 4	1 cup	55	7	201	4	3	0.4	1.0	1.1
442	BERRY BERRY KIX	¾ cup	30	2	120	1	1	0.2	0.5	0.1
443	CAP'N CRUNCH	¾ cup	27	2	107	1	1	0.4	0.3	0.2
444	CAP'N CRUNCH'S CRUNCHBERRIES	¾ cup	26	2	104	1	1	0.3	0.3	0.2
445	CAP'N CRUNCH'S PEANUT BUTTER CRUNCH	¾ cup	27	2	112	2	2	0.5	0.8	0.5
446	CHEERIOS	1 cup	30	3	110	3	2	0.4	0.6	0.2
	CHEX									
447	Corn	1 cup	30	3	113	2	Tr	0.1	0.1	0.2
448	Honey nut	¾ cup	30	2	117	2	1	0.1	0.4	0.2
449	Multi bran	1 cup	49	3	165	4	1	0.2	0.3	0.5
450	Rice	1¼ cup	31	3	117	2	Tr	Tr	Tr	Tr
451	Wheat	1 cup	30	3	104	3	1	0.1	0.1	0.3
452	CINNAMON LIFE	1 cup	50	4	190	4	2	0.3	0.6	0.8
453	CINNAMON TOAST CRUNCH	¾ cup	30	2	124	2	3	0.5	0.9	0.5
454	COCOA KRISPIES	¾ cup	31	2	120	2	1	0.6	0.1	0.1
455	COCOA PUFFS	1 cup	30	2	119	1	1	0.2	0.3	Tr
	Corn Flakes									
456	GENERAL MILLS, TOTAL	1⅓ cup	30	3	112	2	Tr	0.2	0.1	Tr
457	KELLOGG'S	1 cup	28	3	102	2	Tr	0.1	Tr	0.1
458	CORN POPS	1 cup	31	3	118	1	Tr	0.1	0.1	Tr
459	CRISPIX	1 cup	29	3	108	2	Tr	0.1	0.1	0.1
460	Complete Wheat Bran Flakes	¾ cup	29	4	95	3	1	0.1	0.1	0.4
461	FROOT LOOPS	1 cup	30	2	117	1	1	0.4	0.2	0.3
462	FROSTED FLAKES	¾ cup	31	3	119	1	Tr	0.1	Tr	0.1
	FROSTED MINI WHEATS									
463	Regular	1 cup	51	5	173	5	1	0.2	0.1	0.6
464	Bite size	1 cup	55	5	187	5	1	0.2	0.2	0.6
465	GOLDEN GRAHAMS	¾ cup	30	3	116	2	1	0.2	0.3	0.2
466	HONEY FROSTED WHEATIES	¾ cup	30	3	110	2	Tr	0.1	Tr	Tr
467	HONEY NUT CHEERIOS	1 cup	30	2	115	3	1	0.2	0.5	0.2
468	HONEY NUT CLUSTERS	1 cup	55	3	213	5	3	0.4	1.8	0.4
469	KIX	1⅓ cup	30	2	114	2	1	0.2	0.1	Tr
470	LIFE	¾ cup	32	4	121	3	1	0.2	0.4	0.6
471	LUCKY CHARMS	1 cup	30	2	116	2	1	0.2	0.4	0.2
472	NATURE VALLEY Granola	¾ cup	55	4	248	6	10	1.3	6.5	1.9
	100% Natural Cereal									
473	With oats, honey, and raisins	½ cup	51	4	218	5	7	3.2	3.2	0.8
474	With raisins, low fat	½ cup	50	4	195	4	3	0.8	1.3	0.5
475	PRODUCT 19	1 cup	30	3	110	3	Tr	Tr	0.2	0.2
476	Puffed Rice	1 cup	14	3	56	1	Tr	Tr	Tr	Tr
477	Puffed Wheat	1 cup	12	3	44	2	Tr	Tr	Tr	Tr
	Raisin Bran									
478	GENERAL MILLS, TOTAL	1 cup	55	9	178	4	1	0.2	0.2	0.2
479	KELLOGG'S	1 cup	61	8	186	6	1	0.0	0.2	0.8
480	RAISIN NUT BRAN	1 cup	55	5	209	5	4	0.7	1.9	0.5
481	REESE'S PEANUT BUTTER PUFFS	¾ cup	30	2	129	3	3	0.6	1.4	0.6
482	RICE KRISPIES	1¼ cup	33	3	124	2	Tr	0.1	0.1	0.2

Choles-terol (mg)	Carbo-hydrate (g)	Total dietary fiber (g)	Calcium (mg)	Iron (mg)	Potas-sium (mg)	Sodium (mg)	Vitamin A		Thiamin (mg)	Ribo-flavin (mg)	Niacin (mg)	Ascor-bic acid (mg)	Food No.
							(IU)	(RE)					
0	42	3.4	310	4.5	162	323	1,250	375	0.37	0.42	5.0	15	441
0	26	0.2	66	4.5	24	185	750	225	0.38	0.43	5.0	15	442
0	23	0.9	5	4.5	35	208	36	4	0.38	0.42	5.0	0	443
0	22	0.6	7	4.5	37	190	33	5	0.37	0.42	5.0	Tr	444
0	22	0.8	3	4.5	62	204	37	4	0.38	0.42	5.0	0	445
0	23	2.6	55	8.1	89	284	1,250	375	0.38	0.43	5.0	15	446
0	26	0.5	100	9.0	32	289	0	0	0.38	0.00	5.0	6	447
0	26	0.4	102	9.0	27	224	0	0	0.38	0.44	5.0	6	448
0	41	6.4	95	13.7	191	325	0	0	0.32	0.00	4.4	5	449
0	27	0.3	104	9.0	36	291	0	0	0.38	0.02	5.0	6	450
0	24	3.3	60	9.0	116	269	0	0	0.23	0.04	3.0	4	451
0	40	3.0	135	7.5	113	220	16	2	0.63	0.71	8.4	Tr	452
0	24	1.5	42	4.5	44	210	750	225	0.38	0.43	5.0	15	453
0	27	0.4	4	1.8	60	210	750	225	0.37	0.43	5.0	15	454
0	27	0.2	33	4.5	52	181	0	0	0.38	0.43	5.0	15	455
0	26	0.8	237	18.0	34	203	1,250	375	1.50	1.70	20.1	60	456
0	24	0.8	1	8.7	25	298	700	210	0.36	0.39	4.7	14	457
0	28	0.4	2	1.9	23	123	775	233	0.40	0.43	5.2	16	458
0	25	0.6	3	1.8	35	240	750	225	0.38	0.44	5.0	15	459
0	23	4.6	14	8.1	175	226	1,208	363	0.38	0.44	5.0	15	460
0	26	0.6	3	4.2	32	141	703	211	0.39	0.42	5.0	14	461
0	28	0.6	1	4.5	20	200	750	225	0.37	0.43	5.0	15	462
0	42	5.5	18	14.3	170	2	0	0	0.36	0.41	5.0	0	463
0	45	5.9	0	15.4	186	2	0	0	0.33	0.39	4.7	0	464
0	26	0.9	14	4.5	53	275	750	225	0.38	0.43	5.0	15	465
0	26	1.5	8	4.5	56	211	750	225	0.38	0.43	5.0	15	466
0	24	1.6	20	4.5	85	259	750	225	0.38	0.43	5.0	15	467
0	43	4.2	72	4.5	171	239	0	0	0.37	0.42	5.0	9	468
0	26	0.8	44	8.1	41	263	1,250	375	0.38	0.43	5.0	15	469
0	25	2.0	98	9.0	79	174	12	1	0.40	0.45	5.3	0	470
0	25	1.2	32	4.5	54	203	750	225	0.38	0.43	5.0	15	471
0	36	3.5	41	1.7	183	89	0	0	0.17	0.06	0.6	0	472
1	36	3.7	39	1.7	214	11	4	1	0.14	0.09	0.8	Tr	473
1	40	3.0	30	1.3	169	129	9	1	0.15	0.06	0.9	Tr	474
0	25	1.0	3	18.0	41	216	750	225	1.50	1.71	20.0	60	475
0	13	0.2	1	4.4	16	Tr	0	0	0.36	0.25	4.9	0	476
0	10	0.5	3	3.8	42	Tr	0	0	0.31	0.22	4.2	0	477
0	43	5.0	238	18.0	287	240	1,250	375	1.50	1.70	20.0	0	478
0	47	8.2	35	5.0	437	354	832	250	0.43	0.49	5.6	0	479
0	41	5.1	74	4.5	218	246	0	0	0.37	0.42	5.0	0	480
0	23	0.4	21	4.5	62	177	750	225	0.38	0.43	5.0	15	481
0	29	0.4	3	2.0	42	354	825	248	0.43	0.46	5.5	17	482

Table 9. Nutritive Value of the Edible Part of Food

Food No.	Food Description	Measure of edible portion	Weight (g)	Water (%)	Calories (kcal)	Protein (g)	Total fat (g)	Fatty acids		
								Saturated (g)	Mono-unsaturated (g)	Poly-unsaturated (g)

Grain Products (continued)

Breakfast Cereals (continued)
  Ready to eat (continued)

Food No.	Food Description	Measure	Weight (g)	Water (%)	Calories (kcal)	Protein (g)	Total fat (g)	Saturated (g)	Mono-unsat (g)	Poly-unsat (g)
483	RICE KRISPIES TREATS cereal	¾ cup	30	4	120	1	2	0.4	1.0	0.2
484	SHREDDED WHEAT	2 biscuits	46	4	156	5	1	0.1	NA	NA
485	SMACKS	¾ cup	27	3	103	2	1	0.3	0.1	0.2
486	SPECIAL K	1 cup	31	3	115	6	Tr	0.0	0.0	0.2
487	QUAKER Toasted Oatmeal, Honey Nut	1 cup	49	3	191	5	3	0.5	1.2	0.7
488	TOTAL, Whole Grain	¾ cup	30	3	105	3	1	0.2	0.1	0.1
489	TRIX	1 cup	30	2	122	1	2	0.4	0.9	0.3
490	WHEATIES	1 cup	30	3	110	3	1	0.2	0.2	0.2
	Brownies, without icing Commercially prepared									
491	Regular, large (2¾" sq x ⅞")	1 brownie	56	14	227	3	9	2.4	5.0	1.3
492	Fat free, 2" sq	1 brownie	28	12	89	1	Tr	0.2	0.1	Tr
493	Prepared from dry mix, reduced calorie, 2" sq	1 brownie	22	13	84	1	2	1.1	1.0	0.2
494	Buckwheat flour, whole groat	1 cup	120	11	402	15	4	0.8	1.1	1.1
495	Buckwheat groats, roasted (kasha), cooked	1 cup	168	76	155	6	1	0.2	0.3	0.3
	Bulgur									
496	Uncooked	1 cup	140	9	479	17	2	0.3	0.2	0.8
497	Cooked	1 cup	182	78	151	6	Tr	0.1	0.1	0.2
	Cakes, prepared from dry mix									
498	Angelfood (¹⁄₁₂ of 10" dia)	1 piece	50	33	129	3	Tr	Tr	Tr	0.1
499	Yellow, light, with water, egg whites, no frosting (¹⁄₁₂ of 9" dia)	1 piece	69	37	181	3	2	1.1	0.9	0.2
	Cakes, prepared from recipe									
500	Chocolate, without frosting (¹⁄₁₂ of 9" dia)	1 piece	95	24	340	5	14	5.2	5.7	2.6
501	Gingerbread (⅑ of 8" square)	1 piece	74	28	263	3	12	3.1	5.3	3.1
502	Pineapple upside down (⅑ of 8" square)	1 piece	115	32	367	4	14	3.4	6.0	3.8
503	Shortcake, biscuit type (about 3" dia)	1 shortcake	65	28	225	4	9	2.5	3.9	2.4
504	Sponge (¹⁄₁₂ of 16-oz cake)	1 piece	63	29	187	5	3	0.8	1.0	0.4
	White									
505	With coconut frosting (¹⁄₁₂ of 9" dia)	1 piece	112	21	399	5	12	4.4	4.1	2.4
506	Without frosting (¹⁄₁₂ of 9" dia)	1 piece	74	23	264	4	9	2.4	3.9	2.3
	Cakes, commercially prepared									
507	Angelfood (¹⁄₁₂ of 12-oz cake)	1 piece	28	33	72	2	Tr	Tr	Tr	0.1
508	Boston cream (⅙ of pie)	1 piece	92	45	232	2	8	2.2	4.2	0.9
509	Chocolate with chocolate frosting (⅛ of 18-oz cake)	1 piece	64	23	235	3	10	3.1	5.6	1.2
510	Coffeecake, crumb (⅑ of 20-oz cake)	1 piece	63	22	263	4	15	3.7	8.2	2.0
511	Fruitcake	1 piece	43	25	139	1	4	0.5	1.8	1.4
	Pound									
512	Butter (¹⁄₁₂ of 12-oz cake)	1 piece	28	25	109	2	6	3.2	1.7	0.3
513	Fat free (3¼" x 2¾" x ⅝" slice)	1 slice	28	31	79	2	Tr	0.1	Tr	0.1

Choles-terol (mg)	Carbo-hydrate (g)	Total dietary fiber (g)	Calcium (mg)	Iron (mg)	Potas-sium (mg)	Sodium (mg)	Vitamin A (IU)	Vitamin A (RE)	Thiamin (mg)	Ribo-flavin (mg)	Niacin (mg)	Ascor-bic acid (mg)	Food No.
0	26	0.3	2	1.8	19	190	750	225	0.39	0.42	5.0	15	483
0	38	5.3	20	1.4	196	3	0	NA	0.12	0.05	2.6	0	484
0	24	0.9	3	1.8	42	51	750	225	0.38	0.43	5.0	15	485
0	22	1.0	5	8.7	55	250	750	225	0.53	0.59	7.0	15	486
Tr	39	3.3	27	4.5	185	166	500	150	0.37	0.42	5.0	6	487
0	24	2.6	258	18.0	97	199	1,250	375	1.50	1.70	20.1	60	488
0	26	0.7	32	4.5	18	197	750	225	0.38	0.43	5.0	15	489
0	24	2.1	55	8.1	104	222	750	225	0.38	0.43	5.0	15	490
10	36	1.2	16	1.3	83	175	39	3	0.14	0.12	1.0	0	491
0	22	1.0	17	0.7	89	90	1	Tr	0.03	0.04	0.3	Tr	492
0	16	0.8	3	0.3	69	21	0	0	0.02	0.03	0.2	0	493
0	85	12.0	49	4.9	692	13	0	0	0.50	0.23	7.4	0	494
0	33	4.5	12	1.3	148	7	0	0	0.07	0.07	1.6	0	495
0	106	25.6	49	3.4	574	24	0	0	0.32	0.16	7.2	0	496
0	34	8.2	18	1.7	124	9	0	0	0.10	0.05	1.8	0	497
0	29	0.1	42	0.1	68	255	0	0	0.05	0.10	0.1	0	498
0	37	0.6	69	0.6	41	279	6	1	0.06	0.12	0.6	0	499
55	51	1.5	57	1.5	133	299	133	38	0.13	0.20	1.1	Tr	500
24	36	0.7	53	2.1	325	242	36	10	0.14	0.12	1.3	Tr	501
25	58	0.9	138	1.7	129	367	291	75	0.18	0.18	1.4	1	502
2	32	0.8	133	1.7	69	329	47	12	0.20	0.18	1.7	Tr	503
107	36	0.4	26	1.0	89	144	163	49	0.10	0.19	0.8	0	504
1	71	1.1	101	1.3	111	318	43	12	0.14	0.21	1.2	Tr	505
1	42	0.6	96	1.1	70	242	41	12	0.14	0.18	1.1	Tr	506
0	16	0.4	39	0.1	26	210	0	0	0.03	0.14	0.2	0	507
34	39	1.3	21	0.3	36	132	74	21	0.38	0.25	0.2	Tr	508
27	35	1.8	28	1.4	128	214	54	16	0.02	0.09	0.4	Tr	509
20	29	1.3	34	1.2	77	221	70	21	0.13	0.14	1.1	Tr	510
2	26	1.6	14	0.9	66	116	9	2	0.02	0.04	0.3	Tr	511
62	14	0.1	10	0.4	33	111	170	44	0.04	0.06	0.4	0	512
0	17	0.3	12	0.6	31	95	27	8	0.04	0.08	0.2	0	513

Table 9. Nutritive Value of the Edible Part of Food

Food No.	Food Description	Measure of edible portion	Weight (g)	Water (%)	Calories (kcal)	Protein (g)	Total fat (g)	Fatty acids Saturated (g)	Mono- unsaturated (g)	Poly- unsaturated (g)
	Grain Products (continued)									
	Cakes, commercially prepared (continued)									
	Snack cakes									
514	Chocolate, creme filled, with frosting	1 cupcake	50	20	188	2	7	1.4	2.8	2.6
515	Chocolate, with frosting, low fat	1 cupcake	43	23	131	2	2	0.5	0.8	0.2
516	Sponge, creme filled	1 cake	43	20	155	1	5	1.1	1.7	1.4
517	Sponge, individual shortcake	1 shortcake	30	30	87	2	1	0.2	0.3	0.1
	Yellow									
518	With chocolate frosting	1 piece	64	22	243	2	11	3.0	6.1	1.4
519	With vanilla frosting	1 piece	64	22	239	2	9	1.5	3.9	3.3
520	Cheesecake (⅙ of 17-oz cake)	1 piece	80	46	257	4	18	7.9	6.9	1.3
521	Cheese flavor puffs or twists	1 oz	28	2	157	2	10	1.9	5.7	1.3
522	CHEX mix	1 oz (about ⅔ cup)	28	4	120	3	5	1.6	NA	NA
	Cookies									
523	Butter, commercially prepared	1 cookie	5	5	23	Tr	1	0.6	0.3	Tr
	Chocolate chip, medium (2¼"-2½" dia)									
	Commercially prepared									
524	Regular	1 cookie	10	4	48	1	2	0.7	1.2	0.2
525	Reduced fat	1 cookie	10	4	45	1	2	0.4	0.6	0.5
526	From refrigerated dough (spooned from roll)	1 cookie	26	3	128	1	6	2.0	2.9	0.6
527	Prepared from recipe, with margarine	1 cookie	16	6	78	1	5	1.3	1.7	1.3
528	Devil's food, commercially prepared, fat free	1 cookie	16	18	49	1	Tr	0.1	Tr	Tr
529	Fig bar	1 cookie	16	17	56	1	1	0.2	0.5	0.4
	Molasses									
530	Medium	1 cookie	15	6	65	1	2	0.5	1.1	0.3
531	Large (3½"-4" dia)	1 cookie	32	6	138	2	4	1.0	2.3	0.6
	Oatmeal									
	Commercially prepared, with or without raisins									
532	Regular, large	1 cookie	25	6	113	2	5	1.1	2.5	0.6
533	Soft type	1 cookie	15	11	61	1	2	0.5	1.2	0.3
534	Fat free	1 cookie	11	13	36	1	Tr	Tr	Tr	0.1
535	Prepared from recipe, with raisins (2⅝" dia)	1 cookie	15	6	65	1	2	0.5	1.0	0.8
	Peanut butter									
536	Commercially prepared	1 cookie	15	6	72	1	4	0.7	1.9	0.8
537	Prepared from recipe, with margarine (3" dia)	1 cookie	20	6	95	2	5	0.9	2.2	1.4
	Sandwich type, with creme filling									
538	Chocolate cookie	1 cookie	10	2	47	Tr	2	0.4	0.9	0.7
	Vanilla cookie									
539	Oval	1 cookie	15	2	72	1	3	0.4	1.3	1.1
540	Round	1 cookie	10	2	48	Tr	2	0.3	0.8	0.8
	Shortbread, commercially prepared									
541	Plain (1⅝" sq)	1 cookie	8	4	40	Tr	2	0.5	1.1	0.3
	Pecan									
542	Regular (2" dia)	1 cookie	14	3	76	1	5	1.1	2.6	0.6
543	Reduced fat	1 cookie	16	5	73	1	3	0.6	1.6	0.4

Choles-terol (mg)	Carbo-hydrate (g)	Total dietary fiber (g)	Calcium (mg)	Iron (mg)	Potas-sium (mg)	Sodium (mg)	Vitamin A (IU)	Vitamin A (RE)	Thiamin (mg)	Ribo-flavin (mg)	Niacin (mg)	Ascor-bic acid (mg)	Food No.
9	30	0.4	37	1.7	61	213	9	3	0.11	0.15	1.2	0	514
0	29	1.8	15	0.7	96	178	0	0	0.02	0.06	0.3	0	515
7	27	0.2	19	0.5	37	155	7	2	0.07	0.06	0.5	Tr	516
31	18	0.2	21	0.8	30	73	46	14	0.07	0.08	0.6	0	517
35	35	1.2	24	1.3	114	216	70	21	0.08	0.10	0.8	0	518
35	38	0.2	40	0.7	34	220	40	12	0.06	0.04	0.3	0	519
44	20	0.3	41	0.5	72	166	438	117	0.02	0.15	0.2	Tr	520
1	15	0.3	16	0.7	47	298	75	10	0.07	0.10	0.9	Tr	521
0	18	1.6	10	7.0	76	288	41	4	0.44	0.14	4.8	13	522
6	3	Tr	1	0.1	6	18	34	8	0.02	0.02	0.2	0	523
0	7	0.3	3	0.3	14	32	Tr	0	0.02	0.03	0.3	0	524
0	7	0.4	2	0.3	12	38	Tr	0	0.03	0.03	0.3	0	525
7	18	0.4	7	0.7	52	60	15	4	0.04	0.05	0.5	0	526
5	9	0.4	6	0.4	36	58	102	26	0.03	0.03	0.2	Tr	527
0	12	0.3	5	0.4	18	28	Tr	NA	0.01	0.03	0.2	Tr	528
0	11	0.7	10	0.5	33	56	5	1	0.03	0.03	0.3	Tr	529
0	11	0.1	11	1.0	52	69	0	0	0.05	0.04	0.5	0	530
0	24	0.3	24	2.1	111	147	0	0	0.11	0.08	1.0	0	531
0	17	0.7	9	0.6	36	96	5	1	0.07	0.06	0.6	Tr	532
1	10	0.4	14	0.4	20	52	5	1	0.03	0.03	0.3	Tr	533
0	9	0.8	4	0.2	23	33	0	0	0.02	0.03	0.1	0	534
5	10	0.5	15	0.4	36	81	96	25	0.04	0.02	0.2	Tr	535
Tr	9	0.3	5	0.4	25	62	1	Tr	0.03	0.03	0.6	0	536
6	12	0.4	8	0.4	46	104	120	31	0.04	0.04	0.7	Tr	537
0	7	0.3	3	0.4	18	60	Tr	0	0.01	0.02	0.2	0	538
0	11	0.2	4	0.3	14	52	0	0	0.04	0.04	0.4	0	539
0	7	0.2	3	0.2	9	35	0	0	0.03	0.02	0.3	0	540
2	5	0.1	3	0.2	8	36	7	1	0.03	0.03	0.3	0	541
5	8	0.3	4	0.3	10	39	Tr	Tr	0.04	0.03	0.3	0	542
0	11	0.2	8	0.5	15	55	1	Tr	0.05	0.03	0.4	Tr	543

Table 9. Nutritive Value of the Edible Part of Food

Food No.	Food Description	Measure of edible portion	Weight (g)	Water (%)	Calories (kcal)	Protein (g)	Total fat (g)	Fatty acids Saturated (g)	Monounsaturated (g)	Polyunsaturated (g)
	Grain Products (continued)									
	Cookies (continued)									
	Sugar									
544	Commercially prepared	1 cookie	15	5	72	1	3	0.8	1.8	0.4
545	From refrigerated dough	1 cookie	15	5	73	1	3	0.9	2.0	0.4
546	Prepared from recipe, with margarine (3" dia)	1 cookie	14	9	66	1	3	0.7	1.4	1.0
547	Vanilla wafer, lower fat, medium size	1 cookie	4	5	18	Tr	1	0.2	0.3	0.2
	Corn chips									
548	Plain	1 oz	28	1	153	2	9	1.3	2.7	4.7
549	Barbecue flavor	1 oz	28	1	148	2	9	1.3	2.7	4.6
	Cornbread									
550	Prepared from mix, piece 3¾" x 2½" x ¾"	1 piece	60	32	188	4	6	1.6	3.1	0.7
551	Prepared from recipe, with 2% milk, piece 2½" sq x 1½"	1 piece	65	39	173	4	5	1.0	1.2	2.1
	Cornmeal, yellow, dry form									
552	Whole grain	1 cup	122	10	442	10	4	0.6	1.2	2.0
553	Degermed, enriched	1 cup	138	12	505	12	2	0.3	0.6	1.0
554	Self rising, degermed, enriched	1 cup	138	10	490	12	2	0.3	0.6	1.0
555	Cornstarch	1 tbsp	8	8	30	Tr	Tr	Tr	Tr	Tr
	Couscous									
556	Uncooked	1 cup	173	9	650	22	1	0.2	0.2	0.4
557	Cooked	1 cup	157	73	176	6	Tr	Tr	Tr	0.1
	Crackers									
558	Cheese, 1" sq	10 crackers	10	3	50	1	3	0.9	1.2	0.2
	Graham, plain									
559	2½" sq	2 squares	14	4	59	1	1	0.2	0.6	0.5
560	Crushed	1 cup	84	4	355	6	8	1.3	3.4	3.2
561	Melba toast, plain	4 pieces	20	5	78	2	1	0.1	0.2	0.3
562	Rye wafer, whole grain, plain	1 wafer	11	5	37	1	Tr	Tr	Tr	Tr
	Saltine									
563	Square	4 crackers	12	4	52	1	1	0.4	0.8	0.2
564	Oyster type	1 cup	45	4	195	4	5	1.3	2.9	0.8
	Sandwich type									
565	Wheat with cheese	1 sandwich	7	4	33	1	1	0.4	0.8	0.2
566	Cheese with peanut butter	1 sandwich	7	4	34	1	2	0.4	0.8	0.3
	Standard snack type									
567	Bite size	1 cup	62	4	311	5	16	2.3	6.6	5.9
568	Round	4 crackers	12	4	60	1	3	0.5	1.3	1.1
569	Wheat, thin square	4 crackers	8	3	38	1	2	0.4	0.9	0.2
570	Whole wheat	4 crackers	16	3	71	1	3	0.5	0.9	1.1
571	Croissant, butter	1 croissant	57	23	231	5	12	6.6	3.1	0.6
572	Croutons, seasoned	1 cup	40	4	186	4	7	2.1	3.8	0.9
	Danish pastry, enriched									
573	Cheese filled	1 danish	71	31	266	6	16	4.8	8.0	1.8
574	Fruit filled	1 danish	71	27	263	4	13	3.5	7.1	1.7
	Doughnuts									
575	Cake type	1 hole	14	21	59	1	3	0.5	1.3	1.1
576		1 medium	47	21	198	2	11	1.7	4.4	3.7
577	Yeast leavened, glazed	1 hole	13	25	52	1	3	0.8	1.7	0.4
578		1 medium	60	25	242	4	14	3.5	7.7	1.7
579	Eclair, prepared from recipe, 5" x 2" x 1¾"	1 eclair	100	52	262	6	16	4.1	6.5	3.9
	English muffin, plain, enriched									
580	Untoasted	1 muffin	57	42	134	4	1	0.1	0.2	0.5
581	Toasted	1 muffin	52	37	133	4	1	0.1	0.2	0.5

Choles- terol (mg)	Carbo- hydrate (g)	Total dietary fiber (g)	Calcium (mg)	Iron (mg)	Potas- sium (mg)	Sodium (mg)	Vitamin A		Thiamin (mg)	Ribo- flavin (mg)	Niacin (mg)	Ascor- bic acid (mg)	Food No.
							(IU)	(RE)					
8	10	0.1	3	0.3	9	54	14	4	0.03	0.03	0.4	Tr	544
5	10	0.1	14	0.3	24	70	6	2	0.03	0.02	0.4	0	545
4	8	0.2	10	0.3	11	69	135	35	0.04	0.04	0.3	Tr	546
2	3	0.1	2	0.1	4	12	1	Tr	0.01	0.01	0.1	0	547
0	16	1.4	36	0.4	40	179	27	3	0.01	0.04	0.3	0	548
0	16	1.5	37	0.4	67	216	173	17	0.02	0.06	0.5	Tr	549
37	29	1.4	44	1.1	77	467	123	26	0.15	0.16	1.2	Tr	550
26	28	1.9	162	1.6	96	428	180	35	0.19	0.19	1.5	Tr	551
0	94	8.9	7	4.2	350	43	572	57	0.47	0.25	4.4	0	552
0	107	10.2	7	5.7	224	4	570	57	0.99	0.56	6.9	0	553
0	103	9.8	483	6.5	235	1,860	570	57	0.94	0.53	6.3	0	554
0	7	0.1	Tr	Tr	Tr	1	0	0	0.00	0.00	0.0	0	555
0	134	8.7	42	1.9	287	17	0	0	0.28	0.13	6.0	0	556
0	36	2.2	13	0.6	91	8	0	0	0.10	0.04	1.5	0	557
1	6	0.2	15	0.5	15	100	16	3	0.06	0.04	0.5	0	558
0	11	0.4	3	0.5	19	85	0	0	0.03	0.04	0.6	0	559
0	65	2.4	20	3.1	113	508	0	0	0.19	0.26	3.5	0	560
0	15	1.3	19	0.7	40	166	0	0	0.08	0.05	0.8	0	561
0	9	2.5	4	0.7	54	87	1	0	0.05	0.03	0.2	Tr	562
0	9	0.4	14	0.6	15	156	0	0	0.07	0.06	0.6	0	563
0	32	1.4	54	2.4	58	586	0	0	0.25	0.21	2.4	0	564
Tr	4	0.1	18	0.2	30	98	5	1	0.03	0.05	0.3	Tr	565
Tr	4	0.2	6	0.2	17	69	22	2	0.03	0.02	0.5	Tr	566
0	38	1.0	74	2.2	82	525	0	0	0.25	0.21	2.5	0	567
0	7	0.2	14	0.4	16	102	0	0	0.05	0.04	0.5	0	568
0	5	0.4	4	0.4	15	64	0	0	0.04	0.03	0.4	0	569
0	11	1.7	8	0.5	48	105	0	0	0.03	0.02	0.7	0	570
38	26	1.5	21	1.2	67	424	424	106	0.22	0.14	1.2	Tr	571
3	25	2.0	38	1.1	72	495	16	4	0.20	0.17	1.9	0	572
11	26	0.7	25	1.1	70	320	104	32	0.13	0.18	1.4	Tr	573
81	34	1.3	33	1.3	59	251	53	16	0.19	0.16	1.4	3	574
5	7	0.2	6	0.3	18	76	8	2	0.03	0.03	0.3	Tr	575
17	23	0.7	21	0.9	60	257	27	8	0.10	0.11	0.9	Tr	576
1	6	0.2	6	0.3	14	44	2	1	0.05	0.03	0.4	Tr	577
4	27	0.7	26	1.2	65	205	8	2	0.22	0.13	1.7	Tr	578
127	24	0.6	63	1.2	117	337	718	191	0.12	0.27	0.8	Tr	579
0	26	1.5	99	1.4	75	264	0	0	0.25	0.16	2.2	0	580
0	26	1.5	98	1.4	74	262	0	0	0.20	0.14	2.0	Tr	581

Table 9. Nutritive Value of the Edible Part of Food

Food No.	Food Description	Measure of edible portion	Weight (g)	Water (%)	Calories (kcal)	Protein (g)	Total fat (g)	Fatty acids		
								Saturated (g)	Mono-unsaturated (g)	Poly-unsaturated (g)

Grain Products (continued)

Food No.	Food Description	Measure of edible portion	Weight (g)	Water (%)	Calories (kcal)	Protein (g)	Total fat (g)	Saturated (g)	Mono-unsaturated (g)	Poly-unsaturated (g)
	French toast									
582	Prepared from recipe, with 2% milk, fried in margarine	1 slice	65	55	149	5	7	1.8	2.9	1.7
583	Frozen, ready to heat	1 slice	59	53	126	4	4	0.9	1.2	0.7
	Granola bar									
584	Hard, plain	1 bar	28	4	134	3	6	0.7	1.2	3.4
	Soft, uncoated									
585	Chocolate chip	1 bar	28	5	119	2	5	2.9	1.0	0.6
586	Raisin	1 bar	28	6	127	2	5	2.7	0.8	0.9
587	Soft, chocolate-coated, peanut butter	1 bar	28	3	144	3	9	4.8	1.9	0.5
588	Macaroni (elbows), enriched, cooked	1 cup	140	66	197	7	1	0.1	0.1	0.4
589	Matzo, plain	1 matzo	28	4	112	3	Tr	0.1	Tr	0.2
	Muffins									
	Blueberry									
590	Commercially prepared (2¾" dia x 2")	1 muffin	57	38	158	3	4	0.8	1.1	1.4
591	Prepared from mix (2¼" dia x 1¾")	1 muffin	50	36	150	3	4	0.7	1.8	1.5
592	Prepared from recipe, with 2% milk	1 muffin	57	40	162	4	6	1.2	1.5	3.1
593	Bran with raisins, toaster type, toasted	1 muffin	34	27	106	2	3	0.5	0.8	1.7
	Corn									
594	Commercially prepared (2½" dia x 2¼")	1 muffin	57	33	174	3	5	0.8	1.2	1.8
595	Prepared from mix (2¼" dia x 1½")	1 muffin	50	31	161	4	5	1.4	2.6	0.6
596	Oat bran, commercially prepared (2½" dia x 2¼")	1 muffin	57	35	154	4	4	0.6	1.0	2.4
597	Noodles, chow mein, canned	1 cup	45	1	237	4	14	2.0	3.5	7.8
	Noodles (egg noodles), enriched, cooked									
598	Regular	1 cup	160	69	213	8	2	0.5	0.7	0.7
599	Spinach	1 cup	160	69	211	8	3	0.6	0.8	0.6
600	NUTRI GRAIN Cereal Bar, fruit filled	1 bar	37	15	136	2	3	0.6	1.9	0.3
	Oat bran									
601	Uncooked	1 cup	94	7	231	16	7	1.2	2.2	2.6
602	Cooked	1 cup	219	84	88	7	2	0.4	0.6	0.7
603	Oriental snack mix	1 oz (about ¼ cup)	28	3	156	5	7	1.1	2.8	3.0
	Pancakes, plain (4" dia)									
604	Frozen, ready to heat	1 pancake	36	45	82	2	1	0.3	0.4	0.3
605	Prepared from complete mix	1 pancake	38	53	74	2	1	0.2	0.3	0.3
606	Prepared from incomplete mix, with 2% milk, egg and oil	1 pancake	38	53	83	3	3	0.8	0.8	1.1
	Pie crust, baked									
	Standard type									
607	From recipe	1 pie shell	180	10	949	12	62	15.5	27.3	16.4
608	From frozen	1 pie shell	126	11	648	6	41	13.3	19.8	5.1
609	Graham cracker	1 pie shell	239	4	1,181	10	60	12.4	27.2	16.5

Choles-terol (mg)	Carbo-hydrate (g)	Total dietary fiber (g)	Calcium (mg)	Iron (mg)	Potas-sium (mg)	Sodium (mg)	Vitamin A (IU)	Vitamin A (RE)	Thiamin (mg)	Ribo-flavin (mg)	Niacin (mg)	Ascor-bic acid (mg)	Food No.
75	16	0.7	65	1.1	87	311	315	86	0.13	0.21	1.1	Tr	582
48	19	0.7	63	1.3	79	292	110	32	0.16	0.22	1.6	Tr	583
0	18	1.5	17	0.8	95	83	43	4	0.07	0.03	0.4	Tr	584
Tr	20	1.4	26	0.7	96	77	12	1	0.06	0.04	0.3	0	585
Tr	19	1.2	29	0.7	103	80	0	0	0.07	0.05	0.3	0	586
3	15	0.8	31	0.4	96	55	37	10	0.03	0.06	0.9	Tr	587
0	40	1.8	10	2.0	43	1	0	0	0.29	0.14	2.3	0	588
0	24	0.9	4	0.9	32	1	0	0	0.11	0.08	1.1	0	589
17	27	1.5	32	0.9	70	255	19	5	0.08	0.07	0.6	1	590
23	24	0.6	13	0.6	39	219	39	11	0.07	0.16	1.1	1	591
21	23	1.1	108	1.3	70	251	80	22	0.16	0.16	1.3	1	592
3	19	2.8	13	1.0	60	179	58	16	0.07	0.10	0.8	0	593
15	29	1.9	42	1.6	39	297	119	21	0.16	0.19	1.2	0	594
31	25	1.2	38	1.0	66	398	105	23	0.12	0.14	1.1	Tr	595
0	28	2.6	36	2.4	289	224	0	0	0.15	0.05	0.2	0	596
0	26	1.8	9	2.1	54	198	38	4	0.26	0.19	2.7	0	597
53	40	1.8	19	2.5	45	11	32	10	0.30	0.13	2.4	0	598
53	39	3.7	30	1.7	59	19	165	22	0.39	0.20	2.4	0	599
0	27	0.8	15	1.8	73	110	750	227	0.37	0.41	5.0	0	600
0	62	14.5	55	5.1	532	4	0	0	1.10	0.21	0.9	0	601
0	25	5.7	22	1.9	201	2	0	0	0.35	0.07	0.3	0	602
0	15	3.7	15	0.7	93	117	1	0	0.09	0.04	0.9	Tr	603
3	16	0.6	22	1.3	26	183	36	10	0.14	0.17	1.4	Tr	604
5	14	0.5	48	0.6	67	239	12	3	0.08	0.08	0.7	Tr	605
27	11	0.7	82	0.5	76	192	95	27	0.08	0.12	0.5	Tr	606
0	86	3.0	18	5.2	121	976	0	0	0.70	0.50	6.0	0	607
0	62	1.3	26	2.8	139	815	0	0	0.35	0.48	3.1	0	608
0	156	3.6	50	5.2	210	1,365	1,876	483	0.25	0.42	5.1	0	609

Table 9. Nutritive Value of the Edible Part of Food

Food No.	Food Description	Measure of edible portion	Weight (g)	Water (%)	Calories (kcal)	Protein (g)	Total fat (g)	Fatty acids		
								Saturated (g)	Mono-unsaturated (g)	Poly-unsaturated (g)

Grain Products (continued)

Pies
  Commercially prepared (⅙ of 8" dia)

610	Apple	1 piece	117	52	277	2	13	4.4	5.1	2.6
611	Blueberry	1 piece	117	53	271	2	12	2.0	5.0	4.1
612	Cherry	1 piece	117	46	304	2	13	3.0	6.8	2.4
613	Chocolate creme	1 piece	113	44	344	3	22	5.6	12.6	2.7
614	Coconut custard	1 piece	104	49	270	6	14	6.1	5.7	1.2
615	Lemon meringue	1 piece	113	42	303	2	10	2.0	3.0	4.1
616	Pecan	1 piece	113	19	452	5	21	4.0	12.1	3.6
617	Pumpkin	1 piece	109	58	229	4	10	1.9	4.4	3.4

  Prepared from recipe (⅛ of 9" dia)

618	Apple	1 piece	155	47	411	4	19	4.7	8.4	5.2
619	Blueberry	1 piece	147	51	360	4	17	4.3	7.5	4.5
620	Cherry	1 piece	180	46	486	5	22	5.4	9.6	5.8
621	Lemon meringue	1 piece	127	43	362	5	16	4.0	7.1	4.2
622	Pecan	1 piece	122	20	503	6	27	4.9	13.6	7.0
623	Pumpkin	1 piece	155	59	316	7	14	4.9	5.7	2.8
624	Fried, cherry	1 pie	128	38	404	4	21	3.1	9.5	6.9

Popcorn

625	Air popped, unsalted	1 cup	8	4	31	1	Tr	Tr	0.1	0.2
626	Oil popped, salted	1 cup	11	3	55	1	3	0.5	0.9	1.5

  Caramel coated

627	With peanuts	1 cup	42	3	168	3	3	0.4	1.1	1.4
628	Without peanuts	1 cup	35	3	152	1	5	1.3	1.0	1.6
629	Cheese flavor	1 cup	11	3	58	1	4	0.7	1.1	1.7
630	Popcorn cake	1 cake	10	5	38	1	Tr	Tr	0.1	0.1

Pretzels, made with enriched flour

631	Stick, 2¼" long	10 pretzels	3	3	11	Tr	Tr	Tr	Tr	Tr
632	Twisted, regular	10 pretzels	60	3	229	5	2	0.5	0.8	0.7
633	Twisted, dutch, 2¾" x 2⅝"	1 pretzel	16	3	61	1	1	0.1	0.2	0.2

Rice

634	Brown, long grain, cooked	1 cup	195	73	216	5	2	0.4	0.6	0.6

  White, long grain, enriched
    Regular

635	Raw	1 cup	185	12	675	13	1	0.3	0.4	0.3
636	Cooked	1 cup	158	68	205	4	Tr	0.1	0.1	0.1
637	Instant, prepared	1 cup	165	76	162	3	Tr	0.1	0.1	0.1

    Parboiled

638	Raw	1 cup	185	10	686	13	1	0.3	0.3	0.3
639	Cooked	1 cup	175	72	200	4	Tr	0.1	0.1	0.1
640	Wild, cooked	1 cup	164	74	166	7	1	0.1	0.1	0.3
641	Rice cake, brown rice, plain	1 cake	9	6	35	1	Tr	0.1	0.1	0.1
642	RICE KRISPIES Treat Squares	1 bar	22	6	91	1	2	0.3	0.6	1.1

Rolls

643	Dinner	1 roll	28	32	84	2	2	0.5	1.0	0.3
644	Hamburger or hotdog	1 roll	43	34	123	4	2	0.5	0.4	1.1
645	Hard, kaiser	1 roll	57	31	167	6	2	0.3	0.6	1.0

Spaghetti, cooked

646	Enriched	1 cup	140	66	197	7	1	0.1	0.1	0.4
647	Whole wheat	1 cup	140	67	174	7	1	0.1	0.1	0.3

Sweet rolls, cinnamon

648	Commercial, with raisins	1 roll	60	25	223	4	10	1.8	2.9	4.5
649	Refrigerated dough, baked, with frosting	1 roll	30	23	109	2	4	1.0	2.2	0.5

Choles-terol (mg)	Carbo-hydrate (g)	Total dietary fiber (g)	Calcium (mg)	Iron (mg)	Potas-sium (mg)	Sodium (mg)	Vitamin A (IU)	Vitamin A (RE)	Thiamin (mg)	Ribo-flavin (mg)	Niacin (mg)	Ascor-bic acid (mg)	Food No.
0	40	1.9	13	0.5	76	311	145	35	0.03	0.03	0.3	4	610
0	41	1.2	9	0.4	59	380	164	40	0.01	0.04	0.4	3	611
0	47	0.9	14	0.6	95	288	329	63	0.03	0.03	0.2	1	612
6	38	2.3	41	1.2	144	154	0	0	0.04	0.12	0.8	0	613
36	31	1.9	84	0.8	182	348	114	28	0.09	0.15	0.4	1	614
51	53	1.4	63	0.7	101	165	198	59	0.07	0.24	0.7	4	615
36	65	4.0	19	1.2	84	479	198	53	0.10	0.14	0.3	1	616
22	30	2.9	65	0.9	168	307	3,743	405	0.06	0.17	0.2	1	617
0	58	3.6	11	1.7	122	327	90	19	0.23	0.17	1.9	3	618
0	49	3.6	10	1.8	74	272	62	6	0.22	0.19	1.8	1	619
0	69	3.5	18	3.3	139	344	736	86	0.27	0.23	2.3	2	620
67	50	0.7	15	1.3	83	307	203	56	0.15	0.20	1.2	4	621
106	64	2.2	39	1.8	162	320	410	109	0.23	0.22	1.0	Tr	622
65	41	2.9	146	2.0	288	349	11,833	1,212	0.14	0.31	1.2	3	623
0	55	3.3	28	1.6	83	479	220	22	0.18	0.14	1.8	2	624
0	6	1.2	1	0.2	24	Tr	16	2	0.02	0.02	0.2	0	625
0	6	1.1	1	0.3	25	97	17	2	0.01	0.01	0.2	Tr	626
0	34	1.6	28	1.6	149	124	27	3	0.02	0.05	0.8	0	627
2	28	1.8	15	0.6	38	73	18	4	0.02	0.02	0.8	0	628
1	6	1.1	12	0.2	29	98	27	5	0.01	0.03	0.2	Tr	629
0	8	0.3	1	0.2	33	29	7	1	0.01	0.02	0.6	0	630
0	2	0.1	1	0.1	4	51	0	0	0.01	0.02	0.2	0	631
0	48	1.9	22	2.6	88	1,029	0	0	0.28	0.37	3.2	0	632
0	13	0.5	6	0.7	23	274	0	0	0.07	0.10	0.8	0	633
0	45	3.5	20	0.8	84	10	0	0	0.19	0.05	3.0	0	634
0	148	2.4	52	8.0	213	9	0	0	1.07	0.09	7.8	0	635
0	45	0.6	16	1.9	55	2	0	0	0.26	0.02	2.3	0	636
0	35	1.0	13	1.0	7	5	0	0	0.12	0.08	1.5	0	637
0	151	3.1	111	6.6	222	9	0	0	1.10	0.13	6.7	0	638
0	43	0.7	33	2.0	65	5	0	0	0.44	0.03	2.5	0	639
0	35	3.0	5	1.0	166	5	0	0	0.09	0.14	2.1	0	640
0	7	0.4	1	0.1	26	29	4	Tr	0.01	0.01	0.7	0	641
0	18	0.1	1	0.5	9	77	200	60	0.15	0.18	2.0	0	642
Tr	14	0.8	33	0.9	37	146	0	0	0.14	0.09	1.1	Tr	643
0	22	1.2	60	1.4	61	241	0	0	0.21	0.13	1.7	Tr	644
0	30	1.3	54	1.9	62	310	0	0	0.27	0.19	2.4	0	645
0	40	2.4	10	2.0	43	1	0	0	0.29	0.14	2.3	0	646
0	37	6.3	21	1.5	62	4	0	0	0.15	0.06	1.0	0	647
40	31	1.4	43	1.0	67	230	129	38	0.19	0.16	1.4	1	648
0	17	0.6	10	0.8	19	250	1	0	0.12	0.07	1.1	Tr	649

Table 9. Nutritive Value of the Edible Part of Food

Food No.	Food Description	Measure of edible portion	Weight (g)	Water (%)	Calories (kcal)	Protein (g)	Total fat (g)	Fatty acids Saturated (g)	Monounsaturated (g)	Polyunsaturated (g)
	Grain Products (continued)									
650	Taco shell, baked	1 medium	13	6	62	1	3	0.4	1.2	1.1
651	Tapioca, pearl, dry	1 cup	152	11	544	Tr	Tr	Tr	Tr	Tr
	Toaster pastries									
652	Brown sugar cinnamon	1 pastry	50	11	206	3	7	1.8	4.0	0.9
653	Chocolate with frosting	1 pastry	52	13	201	3	5	1.0	2.7	1.1
654	Fruit filled	1 pastry	52	12	204	2	5	0.8	2.2	2.0
655	Low fat	1 pastry	52	12	193	2	3	0.7	1.7	0.5
	Tortilla chips									
	Plain									
656	Regular	1 oz	28	2	142	2	7	1.4	4.4	1.0
657	Low fat, baked	10 chips	14	2	54	2	1	0.1	0.2	0.4
	Nacho flavor									
658	Regular	1 oz	28	2	141	2	7	1.4	4.3	1.0
659	Light, reduced fat	1 oz	28	1	126	2	4	0.8	2.5	0.6
	Tortillas, ready to cook (about 6" dia)									
660	Corn	1 tortilla	26	44	58	1	1	0.1	0.2	0.3
661	Flour	1 tortilla	32	27	104	3	2	0.6	1.2	0.3
	Waffles, plain									
662	Prepared from recipe, 7" dia	1 waffle	75	42	218	6	11	2.1	2.6	5.1
663	Frozen, toasted, 4" dia	1 waffle	33	42	87	2	3	0.5	1.1	0.9
664	Low fat, 4" dia	1 waffle	35	43	83	2	1	0.3	0.4	0.4
	Wheat flours									
	All purpose, enriched									
665	Sifted, spooned	1 cup	115	12	419	12	1	0.2	0.1	0.5
666	Unsifted, spooned	1 cup	125	12	455	13	1	0.2	0.1	0.5
667	Bread, enriched	1 cup	137	13	495	16	2	0.3	0.2	1.0
668	Cake or pastry flour, enriched, unsifted, spooned	1 cup	137	13	496	11	1	0.2	0.1	0.5
669	Self rising, enriched, unsifted, spooned	1 cup	125	11	443	12	1	0.2	0.1	0.5
670	Whole wheat, from hard wheats, stirred, spooned	1 cup	120	10	407	16	2	0.4	0.3	0.9
671	Wheat germ, toasted, plain	1 tbsp	7	6	27	2	1	0.1	0.1	0.5
	Legumes, Nuts, and Seeds									
	Almonds, shelled									
672	Sliced	1 cup	95	5	549	20	48	3.7	30.5	11.6
673	Whole	1 oz (24 nuts)	28	5	164	6	14	1.1	9.1	3.5
	Beans, dry									
	Cooked									
674	Black	1 cup	172	66	227	15	1	0.2	0.1	0.4
675	Great Northern	1 cup	177	69	209	15	1	0.2	Tr	0.3
676	Kidney, red	1 cup	177	67	225	15	1	0.1	0.1	0.5
677	Lima, large	1 cup	188	70	216	15	1	0.2	0.1	0.3
678	Pea (navy)	1 cup	182	63	258	16	1	0.3	0.1	0.4
679	Pinto	1 cup	171	64	234	14	1	0.2	0.2	0.3
	Canned, solids and liquid									
	Baked beans									
680	Plain or vegetarian	1 cup	254	73	236	12	1	0.3	0.1	0.5
681	With frankfurters	1 cup	259	69	368	17	17	6.1	7.3	2.2
682	With pork in tomato sauce	1 cup	253	73	248	13	3	1.0	1.1	0.3
683	With pork in sweet sauce	1 cup	253	71	281	13	4	1.4	1.6	0.5
684	Kidney, red	1 cup	256	77	218	13	1	0.1	0.1	0.5
685	Lima, large	1 cup	241	77	190	12	Tr	0.1	Tr	0.2
686	White	1 cup	262	70	307	19	1	0.2	0.1	0.3

Choles-terol (mg)	Carbo-hydrate (g)	Total dietary fiber (g)	Calcium (mg)	Iron (mg)	Potas-sium (mg)	Sodium (mg)	Vitamin A (IU)	Vitamin A (RE)	Thiamin (mg)	Ribo-flavin (mg)	Niacin (mg)	Ascor-bic acid (mg)	Food No.
0	8	1.0	21	0.3	24	49	0	0	0.03	0.01	0.2	0	650
0	135	1.4	30	2.4	17	2	0	0	0.01	0.00	0.0	0	651
0	34	0.5	17	2.0	57	212	493	112	0.19	0.29	2.3	Tr	652
0	37	0.6	20	1.8	82	203	500	NA	0.16	0.16	2.0	0	653
0	37	1.1	14	1.8	58	218	501	2	0.15	0.19	2.0	Tr	654
0	40	0.8	23	1.8	34	131	494	49	0.15	0.29	2.0	2	655
0	18	1.8	44	0.4	56	150	56	6	0.02	0.05	0.4	0	656
0	11	0.7	22	0.2	37	57	52	6	0.03	0.04	0.1	Tr	657
1	18	1.5	42	0.4	61	201	105	12	0.04	0.05	0.4	1	658
1	20	1.4	45	0.5	77	284	108	12	0.06	0.08	0.1	Tr	659
0	12	1.4	46	0.4	40	42	0	0	0.03	0.02	0.4	0	660
0	18	1.1	40	1.1	42	153	0	0	0.17	0.09	1.1	0	661
52	25	0.7	191	1.7	119	383	171	49	0.20	0.26	1.6	Tr	662
8	13	0.8	77	1.5	42	260	400	120	0.13	0.16	1.5	0	663
9	15	0.4	20	1.9	50	155	506	NA	0.31	0.26	2.6	0	664
0	88	3.1	17	5.3	123	2	0	0	0.90	0.57	6.8	0	665
0	95	3.4	19	5.8	134	3	0	0	0.98	0.62	7.4	0	666
0	99	3.3	21	6.0	137	3	0	0	1.11	0.70	10.3	0	667
0	107	2.3	19	10.0	144	3	0	0	1.22	0.59	9.3	0	668
0	93	3.4	423	5.8	155	1,588	0	0	0.84	0.52	7.3	0	669
0	87	14.6	41	4.7	486	6	0	0	0.54	0.26	7.6	0	670
0	3	0.9	3	0.6	66	Tr	0	0	0.12	0.06	0.4	Tr	671
0	19	11.2	236	4.1	692	1	10	1	0.23	0.77	3.7	0	672
0	6	3.3	70	1.2	206	Tr	3	Tr	0.07	0.23	1.1	0	673
0	41	15.0	46	3.6	611	2	10	2	0.42	0.10	0.9	0	674
0	37	12.4	120	3.8	692	4	2	0	0.28	0.10	1.2	2	675
0	40	13.1	50	5.2	713	4	0	0	0.28	0.10	1.0	2	676
0	39	13.2	32	4.5	955	4	0	0	0.30	0.10	0.8	0	677
0	48	11.6	127	4.5	670	2	4	0	0.37	0.11	1.0	2	678
0	44	14.7	82	4.5	800	3	3	0	0.32	0.16	0.7	4	679
0	52	12.7	127	0.7	752	1,008	434	43	0.39	0.15	1.1	8	680
16	40	17.9	124	4.5	609	1,114	399	39	0.15	0.15	2.3	6	681
18	49	12.1	142	8.3	759	1,113	314	30	0.13	0.12	1.3	8	682
18	53	13.2	154	4.2	673	850	288	28	0.12	0.15	0.9	8	683
0	40	16.4	61	3.2	658	873	0	0	0.27	0.23	1.2	3	684
0	36	11.6	51	4.4	530	810	0	0	0.13	0.08	0.6	0	685
0	57	12.6	191	7.8	1,189	13	0	0	0.25	0.10	0.3	0	686

Table 9. Nutritive Value of the Edible Part of Food

Legumes, Nuts, and Seeds (continued)

Food No.	Food Description	Measure of edible portion	Weight (g)	Water (%)	Calories (kcal)	Protein (g)	Total fat (g)	Fatty acids Saturated (g)	Mono-unsaturated (g)	Poly-unsaturated (g)
	Black eyed peas, dry									
687	Cooked	1 cup	172	70	200	13	1	0.2	0.1	0.4
688	Canned, solids and liquid	1 cup	240	80	185	11	1	0.3	0.1	0.6
689	Brazil nuts, shelled	1 oz (6-8 nuts)	28	3	186	4	19	4.6	6.5	6.8
690	Carob flour	1 cup	103	4	229	5	1	0.1	0.2	0.2
	Cashews, salted									
691	Dry roasted	1 oz	28	2	163	4	13	2.6	7.7	2.2
692	Oil roasted	1 cup	130	4	749	21	63	12.4	36.9	10.6
693		1 oz (18 nuts)	28	4	163	5	14	2.7	8.1	2.3
694	Chestnuts, European, roasted, shelled	1 cup	143	40	350	5	3	0.6	1.1	1.2
	Chickpeas, dry									
695	Cooked	1 cup	164	60	269	15	4	0.4	1.0	1.9
696	Canned, solids and liquid	1 cup	240	70	286	12	3	0.3	0.6	1.2
	Coconut									
	Raw									
697	Piece, about 2" x 2" x ½"	1 piece	45	47	159	1	15	13.4	0.6	0.2
698	Shredded, not packed	1 cup	80	47	283	3	27	23.8	1.1	0.3
699	Dried, sweetened, shredded	1 cup	93	13	466	3	33	29.3	1.4	0.4
700	Hazelnuts (filberts), chopped	1 cup	115	5	722	17	70	5.1	52.5	9.1
701		1 oz	28	5	178	4	17	1.3	12.9	2.2
702	Hummus, commercial	1 tbsp	14	67	23	1	1	0.2	0.6	0.5
703	Lentils, dry, cooked	1 cup	198	70	230	18	1	0.1	0.1	0.3
704	Macadamia nuts, dry roasted, salted	1 cup	134	2	959	10	102	16.0	79.4	2.0
705		1 oz (10-12 nuts)	28	2	203	2	22	3.4	16.8	0.4
	Mixed nuts, with peanuts, salted									
706	Dry roasted	1 oz	28	2	168	5	15	2.0	8.9	3.1
707	Oil roasted	1 oz	28	2	175	5	16	2.5	9.0	3.8
	Peanuts									
	Dry roasted									
708	Salted	1 oz (about 28)	28	2	166	7	14	2.0	7.0	4.4
709	Unsalted	1 cup	146	2	854	35	73	10.1	36.0	22.9
710		1 oz (about 28)	28	2	166	7	14	2.0	7.0	4.4
711	Oil roasted, salted	1 cup	144	2	837	38	71	9.9	35.2	22.4
712		1 oz	28	2	165	7	14	1.9	6.9	4.4
	Peanut butter									
	Regular									
713	Smooth style	1 tbsp	16	1	95	4	8	1.7	3.9	2.2
714	Chunk style	1 tbsp	16	1	94	4	8	1.5	3.8	2.3
715	Reduced fat, smooth	1 tbsp	18	1	94	5	6	1.3	2.9	1.8
716	Peas, split, dry, cooked	1 cup	196	69	231	16	1	0.1	0.2	0.3
717	Pecans, halves	1 cup	108	4	746	10	78	6.7	44.0	23.3
718		1 oz (20 halves)	28	4	196	3	20	1.8	11.6	6.1
719	Pine nuts (pignolia), shelled	1 oz	28	7	160	7	14	2.2	5.4	6.1
720		1 tbsp	9	7	49	2	4	0.7	1.6	1.8
721	Pistachio nuts, dry roasted, with salt, shelled	1 oz (47 nuts)	28	2	161	6	13	1.6	6.8	3.9
722	Pumpkin and squash kernels, roasted, with salt	1 oz (142 seeds)	28	7	148	9	12	2.3	3.7	5.4
723	Refried beans, canned	1 cup	252	76	237	14	3	1.2	1.4	0.4
724	Sesame seeds	1 tbsp	8	5	47	2	4	0.6	1.7	1.9
725	Soybeans, dry, cooked	1 cup	172	63	298	29	15	2.2	3.4	8.7
	Soy products									
726	Miso	1 cup	275	41	567	32	17	2.4	3.7	9.4
727	Soy milk	1 cup	245	93	81	7	5	0.5	0.8	2.0

Choles-terol (mg)	Carbo-hydrate (g)	Total dietary fiber (g)	Calcium (mg)	Iron (mg)	Potas-sium (mg)	Sodium (mg)	Vitamin A (IU)	Vitamin A (RE)	Thiamin (mg)	Ribo-flavin (mg)	Niacin (mg)	Ascor-bic acid (mg)	Food No.
0	36	11.2	41	4.3	478	7	26	3	0.35	0.09	0.9	1	687
0	33	7.9	48	2.3	413	718	31	2	0.18	0.18	0.8	6	688
0	4	1.5	50	1.0	170	1	0	0	0.28	0.03	0.5	Tr	689
0	92	41.0	358	3.0	852	36	14	1	0.05	0.47	2.0	Tr	690
0	9	0.9	13	1.7	160	181	0	0	0.06	0.06	0.4	0	691
0	37	4.9	53	5.3	689	814	0	0	0.55	0.23	2.3	0	692
0	8	1.1	12	1.2	150	177	0	0	0.12	0.05	0.5	0	693
0	76	7.3	41	1.3	847	3	34	3	0.35	0.25	1.9	37	694
0	45	12.5	80	4.7	477	11	44	5	0.19	0.10	0.9	2	695
0	54	10.6	77	3.2	413	718	58	5	0.07	0.08	0.3	9	696
0	7	4.1	6	1.1	160	9	0	0	0.03	0.01	0.2	1	697
0	12	7.2	11	1.9	285	16	0	0	0.05	0.02	0.4	3	698
0	44	4.2	14	1.8	313	244	0	0	0.03	0.02	0.4	1	699
0	19	11.2	131	5.4	782	0	46	5	0.74	0.13	2.1	7	700
0	5	2.7	32	1.3	193	0	11	1	0.18	0.03	0.5	2	701
0	2	0.8	5	0.3	32	53	4	Tr	0.03	0.01	0.1	0	702
0	40	15.6	38	6.6	731	4	16	2	0.33	0.14	2.1	3	703
0	17	10.7	94	3.6	486	355	0	0	0.95	0.12	3.0	1	704
0	4	2.3	20	0.8	103	75	0	0	0.20	0.02	0.6	Tr	705
0	7	2.6	20	1.0	169	190	4	Tr	0.06	0.06	1.3	Tr	706
0	6	2.6	31	0.9	165	185	5	1	0.14	0.06	1.4	Tr	707
0	6	2.3	15	0.6	187	230	0	0	0.12	0.03	3.8	0	708
0	31	11.7	79	3.3	961	9	0	0	0.64	0.14	19.7	0	709
0	6	2.3	15	0.6	187	2	0	0	0.12	0.03	3.8	0	710
0	27	13.2	127	2.6	982	624	0	0	0.36	0.16	20.6	0	711
0	5	2.6	25	0.5	193	123	0	0	0.07	0.03	4.0	0	712
0	3	0.9	6	0.3	107	75	0	0	0.01	0.02	2.1	0	713
0	3	1.1	7	0.3	120	78	0	0	0.02	0.02	2.2	0	714
0	6	0.9	6	0.3	120	97	0	0	0.05	0.01	2.6	0	715
0	41	16.3	27	2.5	710	4	14	2	0.37	0.11	1.7	1	716
0	15	10.4	76	2.7	443	0	83	9	0.71	0.14	1.3	1	717
0	4	2.7	20	0.7	116	0	22	2	0.19	0.04	0.3	Tr	718
0	4	1.3	7	2.6	170	1	8	1	0.23	0.05	1.0	1	719
0	1	0.4	2	0.8	52	Tr	2	Tr	0.07	0.02	0.3	Tr	720
0	8	2.9	31	1.2	293	121	151	15	0.24	0.04	0.4	1	721
0	4	1.1	12	4.2	229	163	108	11	0.06	0.09	0.5	1	722
20	39	13.4	88	4.2	673	753	0	0	0.07	0.04	0.8	15	723
0	1	0.9	10	0.6	33	3	5	1	0.06	0.01	0.4	0	724
0	17	10.3	175	8.8	886	2	15	2	0.27	0.49	0.7	3	725
0	77	14.9	182	7.5	451	10,029	239	25	0.27	0.69	2.4	0	726
0	4	3.2	10	1.4	345	29	78	7	0.39	0.17	0.4	0	727

Table 9. Nutritive Value of the Edible Part of Food

Food No.	Food Description	Measure of edible portion	Weight (g)	Water (%)	Calories (kcal)	Protein (g)	Total fat (g)	Fatty acids Saturated (g)	Monounsaturated (g)	Polyunsaturated (g)
	Legumes, Nuts, and Seeds (continued)									
	Soy products (continued)									
	Tofu									
728	Firm	¼ block	81	84	62	7	4	0.5	0.8	2.0
729	Soft, piece 2½" x 2¾" x 1"	1 piece	120	87	73	8	4	0.6	1.0	2.5
730	Sunflower seed kernels, dry roasted, with salt	¼ cup	32	1	186	6	16	1.7	3.0	10.5
731		1 oz	28	1	165	5	14	1.5	2.7	9.3
732	Tahini	1 tbsp	15	3	89	3	8	1.1	3.0	3.5
733	Walnuts, English	1 cup, chopped	120	4	785	18	78	7.4	10.7	56.6
734		1 oz (14 halves)	28	4	185	4	18	1.7	2.5	13.4
	Meat and Meat Products									
	Beef, cooked									
	Cuts braised, simmered, or pot roasted									
	Relatively fat, such as chuck blade, piece, 2½" x 2½" x ¾"									
735	Lean and fat	3 oz	85	47	293	23	22	8.7	9.4	0.8
736	Lean only	3 oz	85	55	213	26	11	4.3	4.8	0.4
	Relatively lean, such as bottom round, piece, 4⅛" x 2¼" x ½"									
737	Lean and fat	3 oz	85	52	234	24	14	5.4	6.2	0.5
738	Lean only	3 oz	85	58	178	27	7	2.4	3.1	0.3
	Ground beef, broiled									
739	83% lean	3 oz	85	57	218	22	14	5.5	6.1	0.5
740	79% lean	3 oz	85	56	231	21	16	6.2	6.9	0.6
741	73% lean	3 oz	85	54	246	20	18	6.9	7.7	0.7
742	Liver, fried, slice, 6½" x 2⅜" x ⅜"	3 oz	85	56	184	23	7	2.3	1.4	1.5
	Roast, oven cooked, no liquid added									
	Relatively fat, such as rib, 2 pieces, 4⅛" x 2¼" x ¼"									
743	Lean and fat	3 oz	85	47	304	19	25	9.9	10.6	0.9
744	Lean only	3 oz	85	59	195	23	11	4.2	4.5	0.3
	Relatively lean, such as eye of round, 2 pieces, 2½" x 2½" x ⅜"									
745	Lean and fat	3 oz	85	59	195	23	11	4.2	4.7	0.4
746	Lean only	3 oz	85	65	143	25	4	1.5	1.8	0.1
	Steak, sirloin, broiled, piece, 2½" x 2½" x ¾"									
747	Lean and fat	3 oz	85	57	219	24	13	5.2	5.6	0.5
748	Lean only	3 oz	85	62	166	26	6	2.4	2.6	0.2
749	Beef, canned, corned	3 oz	85	58	213	23	13	5.3	5.1	0.5
750	Beef, dried, chipped	1 oz	28	57	47	8	1	0.5	0.5	0.1
	Lamb, cooked									
	Chops									
	Arm, braised									
751	Lean and fat	3 oz	85	44	294	26	20	8.4	8.7	1.5
752	Lean only	3 oz	85	49	237	30	12	4.3	5.2	0.8
	Loin, broiled									
753	Lean and fat	3 oz	85	52	269	21	20	8.4	8.2	1.4
754	Lean only	3 oz	85	61	184	25	8	3.0	3.6	0.5

Choles-terol (mg)	Carbo-hydrate (g)	Total dietary fiber (g)	Calcium (mg)	Iron (mg)	Potas-sium (mg)	Sodium (mg)	Vitamin A		Thiamin (mg)	Ribo-flavin (mg)	Niacin (mg)	Ascor-bic acid (mg)	Food No.
							(IU)	(RE)					
0	2	0.3	131	1.2	143	6	6	1	0.08	0.08	Tr	Tr	728
0	2	0.2	133	1.3	144	10	8	1	0.06	0.04	0.6	Tr	729
0	8	2.9	22	1.2	272	250	0	0	0.03	0.08	2.3	Tr	730
0	7	2.6	20	1.1	241	221	0	0	0.03	0.07	2.0	Tr	731
0	3	1.4	64	1.3	62	17	10	1	0.18	0.07	0.8	0	732
0	16	8.0	125	3.5	529	2	49	5	0.41	0.18	2.3	2	733
0	4	1.9	29	0.8	125	1	12	1	0.10	0.04	0.5	Tr	734
88	0	0.0	11	2.6	196	54	0	0	0.06	0.20	2.1	0	735
90	0	0.0	11	3.1	224	60	0	0	0.07	0.24	2.3	0	736
82	0	0.0	5	2.7	240	43	0	0	0.06	0.20	3.2	0	737
82	0	0.0	4	2.9	262	43	0	0	0.06	0.22	3.5	0	738
71	0	0.0	6	2.0	266	60	0	0	0.05	0.23	4.2	0	739
74	0	0.0	9	1.8	256	65	0	0	0.04	0.18	4.4	0	740
77	0	0.0	9	2.1	248	71	0	0	0.03	0.16	4.9	0	741
410	7	0.0	9	5.3	309	90	30,689	9,120	0.18	3.52	12.3	20	742
71	0	0.0	9	2.0	256	54	0	0	0.06	0.14	2.9	0	743
68	0	0.0	9	2.4	318	61	0	0	0.07	0.18	3.5	0	744
61	0	0.0	5	1.6	308	50	0	0	0.07	0.14	3.0	0	745
59	0	0.0	4	1.7	336	53	0	0	0.08	0.14	3.2	0	746
77	0	0.0	9	2.6	311	54	0	0	0.09	0.23	3.3	0	747
76	0	0.0	9	2.9	343	56	0	0	0.11	0.25	3.6	0	748
73	0	0.0	10	1.8	116	855	0	0	0.02	0.12	2.1	0	749
12	Tr	0.0	2	1.3	126	984	0	0	0.02	0.06	1.5	0	750
102	0	0.0	21	2.0	260	61	0	0	0.06	0.21	5.7	0	751
103	0	0.0	22	2.3	287	65	0	0	0.06	0.23	5.4	0	752
85	0	0.0	17	1.5	278	65	0	0	0.09	0.21	6.0	0	753
81	0	0.0	16	1.7	320	71	0	0	0.09	0.24	5.8	0	754

Table 9. Nutritive Value of the Edible Part of Food

Meat and Meat Products (continued)

Food No.	Food Description	Measure of edible portion	Weight (g)	Water (%)	Calories (kcal)	Protein (g)	Total fat (g)	Fatty acids Saturated (g)	Mono-unsaturated (g)	Poly-unsaturated (g)
	Lamb (continued)									
	Leg, roasted, 2 pieces, 4⅛" x 2¼" x ¼"									
755	Lean and fat	3 oz	85	57	219	22	14	5.9	5.9	1.0
756	Lean only	3 oz	85	64	162	24	7	2.3	2.9	0.4
	Rib, roasted, 3 pieces, 2½" x 2½" x ¼"									
757	Lean and fat	3 oz	85	48	305	18	25	10.9	10.6	1.8
758	Lean only	3 oz	85	60	197	22	11	4.0	5.0	0.7
	Pork, cured, cooked									
	Bacon									
759	Regular	3 medium slices	19	13	109	6	9	3.3	4.5	1.1
760	Canadian style (6 slices per 6-oz pkg)	2 slices	47	62	86	11	4	1.3	1.9	0.4
	Ham, light cure, roasted, 2 pieces, 4⅛" x 2¼" x ¼"									
761	Lean and fat	3 oz	85	58	207	18	14	5.1	6.7	1.5
762	Lean only	3 oz	85	66	133	21	5	1.6	2.2	0.5
763	Ham, canned, roasted, 2 pieces, 4⅛" x 2¼" x ¼"	3 oz	85	67	142	18	7	2.4	3.5	0.8
	Pork, fresh, cooked									
	Chop, loin (cut 3 per lb with bone)									
	Broiled									
764	Lean and fat	3 oz	85	58	204	24	11	4.1	5.0	0.8
765	Lean only	3 oz	85	61	172	26	7	2.5	3.1	0.5
	Pan fried									
766	Lean and fat	3 oz	85	53	235	25	14	5.1	6.0	1.6
767	Lean only	3 oz	85	57	197	27	9	3.1	3.8	1.1
	Ham (leg), roasted, piece, 2½" x 2½" x ¾"									
768	Lean and fat	3 oz	85	55	232	23	15	5.5	6.7	1.4
769	Lean only	3 oz	85	61	179	25	8	2.8	3.8	0.7
	Rib roast, piece, 2½" x 2½" x ¾"									
770	Lean and fat	3 oz	85	56	217	23	13	5.0	5.9	1.1
771	Lean only	3 oz	85	59	190	24	9	3.7	4.5	0.7
	Ribs, lean and fat, cooked									
772	Backribs, roasted	3 oz	85	45	315	21	25	9.3	11.4	2.0
773	Country style, braised	3 oz	85	54	252	20	18	6.8	7.9	1.6
774	Spareribs, braised	3 oz	85	40	337	25	26	9.5	11.5	2.3
	Shoulder cut, braised, 3 pieces, 2½" x 2½" x ¼"									
775	Lean and fat	3 oz	85	48	280	24	20	7.2	8.8	1.9
776	Lean only	3 oz	85	54	211	27	10	3.5	4.9	1.0
	Sausages and luncheon meats									
777	Bologna, beef and pork (8 slices per 8-oz pkg)	2 slices	57	54	180	7	16	6.1	7.6	1.4
778	Braunschweiger (6 slices per 6-oz pkg)	2 slices	57	48	205	8	18	6.2	8.5	2.1
779	Brown and serve, cooked, link, 4" x ⅞" raw	2 links	26	45	103	4	9	3.4	4.5	1.0
	Canned, minced luncheon meat									
780	Pork, ham, and chicken, reduced sodium (7 slices per 7-oz can)	2 slices	57	56	172	7	15	5.1	7.1	1.5
781	Pork with ham (12 slices per 12-oz can)	2 slices	57	52	188	8	17	5.7	7.7	1.2
782	Pork and chicken (12 slices per 12-oz can)	2 slices	57	64	117	9	8	2.7	3.8	0.8

Choles-terol (mg)	Carbo-hydrate (g)	Total dietary fiber (g)	Calcium (mg)	Iron (mg)	Potas-sium (mg)	Sodium (mg)	Vitamin A		Thiamin (mg)	Ribo-flavin (mg)	Niacin (mg)	Ascor-bic acid (mg)	Food No.
							(IU)	(RE)					
79	0	0.0	9	1.7	266	56	0	0	0.09	0.23	5.6	0	755
76	0	0.0	7	1.8	287	58	0	0	0.09	0.25	5.4	0	756
82	0	0.0	19	1.4	230	62	0	0	0.08	0.18	5.7	0	757
75	0	0.0	18	1.5	268	69	0	0	0.08	0.20	5.2	0	758
16	Tr	0.0	2	0.3	92	303	0	0	0.13	0.05	1.4	0	759
27	1	0.0	5	0.4	181	719	0	0	0.38	0.09	3.2	0	760
53	0	0.0	6	0.7	243	1,009	0	0	0.51	0.19	3.8	0	761
47	0	0.0	6	0.8	269	1,128	0	0	0.58	0.22	4.3	0	762
35	Tr	0.0	6	0.9	298	908	0	0	0.82	0.21	4.3	0	763
70	0	0.0	28	0.7	304	49	8	3	0.91	0.24	4.5	Tr	764
70	0	0.0	26	0.7	319	51	7	2	0.98	0.26	4.7	Tr	765
78	0	0.0	23	0.8	361	68	7	2	0.97	0.26	4.8	1	766
78	0	0.0	20	0.8	382	73	7	2	1.06	0.28	5.1	1	767
80	0	0.0	12	0.9	299	51	9	3	0.54	0.27	3.9	Tr	768
80	0	0.0	6	1.0	317	54	8	3	0.59	0.30	4.2	Tr	769
62	0	0.0	24	0.8	358	39	5	2	0.62	0.26	5.2	Tr	770
60	0	0.0	22	0.8	371	40	5	2	0.64	0.27	5.5	Tr	771
100	0	0.0	38	1.2	268	86	8	3	0.36	0.17	3.0	Tr	772
74	0	0.0	25	1.0	279	50	7	2	0.43	0.22	3.3	1	773
103	0	0.0	40	1.6	272	79	9	3	0.35	0.32	4.7	0	774
93	0	0.0	15	1.4	314	75	8	3	0.46	0.26	4.4	Tr	775
97	0	0.0	7	1.7	344	87	7	2	0.51	0.31	5.0	Tr	776
31	2	0.0	7	0.9	103	581	0	0	0.10	0.08	1.5	0	777
89	2	0.0	5	5.3	113	652	8,009	2,405	0.14	0.87	4.8	0	778
18	1	0.0	3	0.3	49	209	0	0	0.09	0.04	0.9	0	779
43	1	0.0	0	0.4	321	539	0	0	0.15	0.10	1.8	18	780
40	1	0.0	0	0.4	233	758	0	0	0.18	0.10	2.0	0	781
43	1	0.0	0	0.7	352	539	0	0	0.10	0.12	2.0	18	782

Table 9. Nutritive Value of the Edible Part of Food

Food No.	Food Description	Measure of edible portion	Weight (g)	Water (%)	Calories (kcal)	Protein (g)	Total fat (g)	Fatty acids Saturated (g)	Monounsaturated (g)	Polyunsaturated (g)
Meat and Meat Products (continued)										
	Sausages and luncheon meats (continued)									
783	Chopped ham (8 slices per 6-oz pkg)	2 slices	21	64	48	4	4	1.2	1.7	0.4
	Cooked ham (8 slices per 8-oz pkg)									
784	Regular	2 slices	57	65	104	10	6	1.9	2.8	0.7
785	Extra lean	2 slices	57	71	75	11	3	0.9	1.3	0.3
	Frankfurter (10 per 1-lb pkg), heated									
786	Beef and pork	1 frank	45	54	144	5	13	4.8	6.2	1.2
787	Beef	1 frank	45	55	142	5	13	5.4	6.1	0.6
	Pork sausage, fresh, cooked									
788	Link (4" x ⅞" raw)	2 links	26	45	96	5	8	2.8	3.6	1.0
789	Patty (3⅞" x ¼" raw)	1 patty	27	45	100	5	8	2.9	3.8	1.0
	Salami, beef and pork									
790	Cooked type (8 slices per 8-oz pkg)	2 slices	57	60	143	8	11	4.6	5.2	1.2
791	Dry type, slice, 3⅛" x 1/16"	2 slices	20	35	84	5	7	2.4	3.4	0.6
792	Sandwich spread (pork, beef)	1 tbsp	15	60	35	1	3	0.9	1.1	0.4
793	Vienna sausage (7 per 4-oz can)	1 sausage	16	60	45	2	4	1.5	2.0	0.3
	Veal, lean and fat, cooked									
794	Cutlet, braised, 4⅛" x 2¼" x ½"	3 oz	85	55	179	31	5	2.2	2.0	0.4
795	Rib, roasted, 2 pieces, 4⅛" x 2¼" x ¼"	3 oz	85	60	194	20	12	4.6	4.6	0.8
Mixed Dishes and Fast Foods										
	Mixed dishes									
796	Beef macaroni, frozen, HEALTHY CHOICE	1 package	240	78	211	14	2	0.7	1.2	0.3
797	Beef stew, canned	1 cup	232	82	218	11	12	5.2	5.5	0.5
798	Chicken pot pie, frozen	1 small pie	217	60	484	13	29	9.7	12.5	4.5
799	Chili con carne with beans, canned	1 cup	222	74	255	20	8	2.1	2.2	1.4
800	Macaroni and cheese, canned, made with corn oil	1 cup	252	82	199	8	6	3.0	NA	1.3
801	Meatless burger crumbles, MORNINGSTAR FARMS	1 cup	110	60	231	22	13	3.3	4.6	4.9
802	Meatless burger patty, frozen, MORNINGSTAR FARMS	1 patty	85	71	91	14	1	0.1	0.3	0.2
803	Pasta with meatballs in tomato sauce, canned	1 cup	252	78	260	11	10	4.0	4.2	0.6
804	Spaghetti bolognese (meat sauce), frozen, HEALTHY CHOICE	1 package	283	78	255	14	3	1.0	0.9	0.9
805	Spaghetti in tomato sauce with cheese, canned	1 cup	252	80	192	6	2	0.7	0.3	0.3
806	Spinach souffle, home-prepared	1 cup	136	74	219	11	18	7.1	6.8	3.1
807	Tortellini, pasta with cheese filling, frozen	¾ cup (yields 1 cup cooked)	81	31	249	11	6	2.9	1.7	0.4

Choles-terol (mg)	Carbo-hydrate (g)	Total dietary fiber (g)	Calcium (mg)	Iron (mg)	Potas-sium (mg)	Sodium (mg)	Vitamin A (IU)	(RE)	Thiamin (mg)	Ribo-flavin (mg)	Niacin (mg)	Ascor-bic acid (mg)	Food No.
11	0	0.0	1	0.2	67	288	0	0	0.13	0.04	0.8	0	783
32	2	0.0	4	0.6	189	751	0	0	0.49	0.14	3.0	0	784
27	1	0.0	4	0.4	200	815	0	0	0.53	0.13	2.8	0	785
23	1	0.0	5	0.5	75	504	0	0	0.09	0.05	1.2	0	786
27	1	0.0	9	0.6	75	462	0	0	0.02	0.05	1.1	0	787
22	Tr	0.0	8	0.3	94	336	0	0	0.19	0.07	1.2	1	788
22	Tr	0.0	9	0.3	97	349	0	0	0.20	0.07	1.2	1	789
37	1	0.0	7	1.5	113	607	0	0	0.14	0.21	2.0	0	790
16	1	0.0	2	0.3	76	372	0	0	0.12	0.06	1.0	0	791
6	2	Tr	2	0.1	17	152	13	1	0.03	0.02	0.3	0	792
8	Tr	0.0	2	0.1	16	152	0	0	0.01	0.02	0.3	0	793
114	0	0.0	7	1.1	326	57	0	0	0.05	0.30	9.0	0	794
94	0	0.0	9	0.8	251	78	0	0	0.04	0.23	5.9	0	795
14	33	4.6	46	2.7	365	444	514	50	0.28	0.16	3.1	58	796
37	16	3.5	28	1.6	404	947	3,860	494	0.17	0.14	2.9	10	797
41	43	1.7	33	2.1	256	857	2,285	343	0.25	0.36	4.1	2	798
24	24	8.2	67	3.3	608	1,032	884	93	0.15	0.15	2.1	1	799
8	29	3.0	113	2.0	123	1,058	713	NA	0.28	0.25	2.5	0	800
0	7	5.1	79	6.4	178	476	0	0	9.92	0.35	3.0	0	801
0	8	4.3	87	2.9	434	383	0	0	0.26	0.55	4.1	0	802
20	31	6.8	28	2.3	416	1,053	920	93	0.19	0.16	3.3	8	803
17	43	5.1	51	3.5	408	473	492	48	0.35	3.77	0.5	15	804
8	39	7.8	40	2.8	305	963	932	58	0.35	0.28	4.5	10	805
184	3	NA	230	1.3	201	763	3,461	675	0.09	0.30	0.5	3	806
34	38	1.5	123	1.2	72	279	50	13	0.25	0.25	2.2	0	807

Table 9. Nutritive Value of the Edible Part of Food

Food No.	Food Description	Measure of edible portion	Weight (g)	Water (%)	Calories (kcal)	Protein (g)	Total fat (g)	Fatty acids Saturated (g)	Fatty acids Mono-unsaturated (g)	Fatty acids Poly-unsaturated (g)

Mixed Dishes and Fast Foods (continued)

Fast foods
  Breakfast items

Food No.	Food Description	Measure	Weight	Water	Calories	Protein	Total fat	Sat	Mono	Poly
808	Biscuit with egg and sausage	1 biscuit	180	43	581	19	39	15.0	16.4	4.4
809	Croissant with egg, cheese, bacon	1 croissant	129	44	413	16	28	15.4	9.2	1.8
	Danish pastry									
810	Cheese filled	1 pastry	91	34	353	6	25	5.1	15.6	2.4
811	Fruit filled	1 pastry	94	29	335	5	16	3.3	10.1	1.6
812	English muffin with egg, cheese, Canadian bacon	1 muffin	137	57	289	17	13	4.7	4.7	1.6
813	French toast with butter	2 slices	135	51	356	10	19	7.7	7.1	2.4
814	French toast sticks	5 sticks	141	30	513	8	29	4.7	12.6	9.9
815	Hashed brown potatoes	½ cup	72	60	151	2	9	4.3	3.9	0.5
816	Pancakes with butter, syrup	2 pancakes	232	50	520	8	14	5.9	5.3	2.0
	Burrito									
817	With beans and cheese	1 burrito	93	54	189	8	6	3.4	1.2	0.9
818	With beans and meat	1 burrito	116	52	255	11	9	4.2	3.5	0.6
	Cheeseburger									
	Regular size, with condiments									
819	Double patty with mayo type dressing, vegetables	1 sandwich	166	51	417	21	21	8.7	7.8	2.7
820	Single patty	1 sandwich	113	48	295	16	14	6.3	5.3	1.1
	Regular size, plain									
821	Double patty	1 sandwich	155	42	457	28	28	13.0	11.0	1.9
822	Double patty with 3-piece bun	1 sandwich	160	43	461	22	22	9.5	8.3	1.8
823	Single patty	1 sandwich	102	37	319	15	15	6.5	5.8	1.5
	Large, with condiments									
824	Single patty with mayo type dressing, vegetables	1 sandwich	219	53	563	28	33	15.0	12.6	2.0
825	Single patty with bacon	1 sandwich	195	44	608	32	37	16.2	14.5	2.7
826	Chicken fillet (breaded and fried) sandwich, plain	1 sandwich	182	47	515	24	29	8.5	10.4	8.4
	Chicken, fried. See Poultry and Poultry Products.									
827	Chicken pieces, boneless, breaded and fried, plain	6 pieces	106	47	319	18	21	4.7	10.5	4.6
828	Chili con carne	1 cup	253	77	256	25	8	3.4	3.4	0.5
829	Chimichanga with beef	1 chimichanga	174	51	425	20	20	8.5	8.1	1.1
830	Coleslaw	¾ cup	99	74	147	1	11	1.6	2.4	6.4
	Desserts									
831	Ice milk, soft, vanilla, in cone	1 cone	103	65	164	4	6	3.5	1.8	0.4
832	Pie, fried, with fruit filling (5" x 3¾")	1 pie	128	38	404	4	21	3.1	9.5	6.9
833	Sundae, hot fudge	1 sundae	158	60	284	6	9	5.0	2.3	0.8
834	Enchilada with cheese	1 enchilada	163	63	319	10	19	10.6	6.3	0.8
835	Fish sandwich, with tartar sauce and cheese	1 sandwich	183	45	523	21	29	8.1	8.9	9.4
836	French fries	1 small	85	35	291	4	16	3.3	9.0	2.7
837		1 medium	134	35	458	6	25	5.2	14.3	4.2
838		1 large	169	35	578	7	31	6.5	18.0	5.3
839	Frijoles (refried beans, chili sauce, cheese)	1 cup	167	69	225	11	8	4.1	2.6	0.7

Choles-terol (mg)	Carbo-hydrate (g)	Total dietary fiber (g)	Calcium (mg)	Iron (mg)	Potas-sium (mg)	Sodium (mg)	Vitamin A		Thiamin (mg)	Ribo-flavin (mg)	Niacin (mg)	Ascor-bic acid (mg)	Food No.
							(IU)	(RE)					
302	41	0.9	155	4.0	320	1,141	635	164	0.50	0.45	3.6	0	808
215	24	NA	151	2.2	201	889	472	120	0.35	0.34	2.2	2	809
20	29	NA	70	1.8	116	319	155	43	0.26	0.21	2.5	3	810
19	45	NA	22	1.4	110	333	86	24	0.29	0.21	1.8	2	811
234	27	1.5	151	2.4	199	729	586	156	0.49	0.45	3.3	2	812
116	36	NA	73	1.9	177	513	473	146	0.58	0.50	3.9	Tr	813
75	58	2.7	78	3.0	127	499	45	13	0.23	0.25	3.0	0	814
9	16	NA	7	0.5	267	290	18	3	0.08	0.01	1.1	5	815
58	91	NA	128	2.6	251	1,104	281	70	0.39	0.56	3.4	3	816
14	27	NA	107	1.1	248	583	625	119	0.11	0.35	1.8	1	817
24	33	NA	53	2.5	329	670	319	32	0.27	0.42	2.7	1	818
60	35	NA	171	3.4	335	1,051	398	65	0.35	0.28	8.1	2	819
37	27	NA	111	2.4	223	616	462	94	0.25	0.23	3.7	2	820
110	22	NA	233	3.4	308	636	332	79	0.25	0.37	6.0	0	821
80	44	NA	224	3.7	285	891	277	66	0.34	0.38	6.0	0	822
50	32	NA	141	2.4	164	500	153	37	0.40	0.40	3.7	0	823
88	38	NA	206	4.7	445	1,108	613	129	0.39	0.46	7.4	8	824
111	37	NA	162	4.7	332	1,043	406	80	0.31	0.41	6.6	2	825
60	39	NA	60	4.7	353	957	100	31	0.33	0.24	6.8	9	826
61	15	0.0	14	0.9	305	513	0	0	0.12	0.16	7.5	0	827
134	22	NA	68	5.2	691	1,007	1,662	167	0.13	1.14	2.5	2	828
9	43	NA	63	4.5	586	910	146	16	0.49	0.64	5.8	5	829
5	13	NA	34	0.7	177	267	338	50	0.04	0.03	0.1	8	830
28	24	0.1	153	0.2	169	92	211	52	0.05	0.26	0.3	1	831
0	55	3.3	28	1.6	83	479	35	4	0.18	0.14	1.8	2	832
21	48	0.0	207	0.6	395	182	221	57	0.06	0.30	1.1	2	833
44	29	NA	324	1.3	240	784	1,161	186	0.08	0.42	1.9	1	834
68	48	NA	185	3.5	353	939	432	97	0.46	0.42	4.2	3	835
0	34	3.0	12	0.7	586	168	0	0	0.07	0.03	2.4	10	836
0	53	4.7	19	1.0	923	265	0	0	0.11	0.05	3.8	16	837
0	67	5.9	24	1.3	1,164	335	0	0	0.14	0.07	4.8	20	838
37	29	NA	189	2.2	605	882	456	70	0.13	0.33	1.5	2	839

Table 9. Nutritive Value of the Edible Part of Food

Food No.	Food Description	Measure of edible portion	Weight (g)	Water (%)	Calories (kcal)	Protein (g)	Total fat (g)	Fatty acids Saturated (g)	Mono-unsaturated (g)	Poly-unsaturated (g)
	Mixed Dishes and Fast Foods (continued)									
	Fast foods (continued)									
	Hamburger									
	Regular size, with condiments									
840	Double patty	1 sandwich	215	51	576	32	32	12.0	14.1	2.8
841	Single patty	1 sandwich	106	45	272	12	10	3.6	3.4	1.0
	Large, with condiments, mayo type dressing, and vegetables									
842	Double patty	1 sandwich	226	54	540	34	27	10.5	10.3	2.8
843	Single patty	1 sandwich	218	56	512	26	27	10.4	11.4	2.2
	Hot dog									
844	Plain	1 sandwich	98	54	242	10	15	5.1	6.9	1.7
845	With chili	1 sandwich	114	48	296	14	13	4.9	6.6	1.2
846	With corn flour coating (corndog)	1 corndog	175	47	460	17	19	5.2	9.1	3.5
847	Hush puppies	5 pieces	78	32	257	5	12	2.7	7.8	0.4
848	Mashed potatoes	⅓ cup	80	79	66	2	1	0.4	0.3	0.2
849	Nachos, with cheese sauce	6-8 nachos	113	40	346	9	19	7.8	8.0	2.2
850	Onion rings, breaded and fried	8-9 rings	83	37	276	4	16	7.0	6.7	0.7
	Pizza (slice = ⅛ of 12" pizza)									
851	Cheese	1 slice	63	48	140	8	3	1.5	1.0	0.5
852	Meat and vegetables	1 slice	79	48	184	13	5	1.5	2.5	0.9
853	Pepperoni	1 slice	71	47	181	10	7	2.2	3.1	1.2
854	Roast beef sandwich, plain	1 sandwich	139	49	346	22	14	3.6	6.8	1.7
855	Salad, tossed, with chicken, no dressing	1½ cups	218	87	105	17	2	0.6	0.7	0.6
856	Salad, tossed, with egg, cheese, no dressing	1½ cups	217	90	102	9	6	3.0	1.8	0.5
	Shake									
857	Chocolate	16 fl oz	333	72	423	11	12	7.7	3.6	0.5
858	Vanilla	16 fl oz	333	75	370	12	10	6.2	2.9	0.4
859	Shrimp, breaded and fried	6-8 shrimp	164	48	454	19	25	5.4	17.4	0.6
	Submarine sandwich (6" long), with oil and vinegar									
860	Cold cuts (with lettuce, cheese, salami, ham, tomato, onion)	1 sandwich	228	58	456	22	19	6.8	8.2	2.3
861	Roast beef (with tomato, lettuce, mayo)	1 sandwich	216	59	410	29	13	7.1	1.8	2.6
862	Tuna salad (with mayo, lettuce)	1 sandwich	256	54	584	30	28	5.3	13.4	7.3
863	Taco, beef	1 small	171	58	369	21	21	11.4	6.6	1.0
864		1 large	263	58	568	32	32	17.5	10.1	1.5
865	Taco salad (with ground beef, cheese, taco shell)	1½ cups	198	72	279	13	15	6.8	5.2	1.7
	Tostada (with cheese, tomato, lettuce)									
866	With beans and beef	1 tostada	225	70	333	16	17	11.5	3.5	0.6
867	With guacamole	1 tostada	131	73	181	6	12	5.0	4.3	1.5

Choles-terol (mg)	Carbo-hydrate (g)	Total dietary fiber (g)	Calcium (mg)	Iron (mg)	Potas-sium (mg)	Sodium (mg)	Vitamin A (IU)	Vitamin A (RE)	Thiamin (mg)	Ribo-flavin (mg)	Niacin (mg)	Ascor-bic acid (mg)	Food No.
103	39	NA	92	5.5	527	742	54	4	0.34	0.41	6.7	1	840
30	34	2.3	126	2.7	251	534	74	10	0.29	0.24	3.9	2	841
122	40	NA	102	5.9	570	791	102	11	0.36	0.38	7.6	1	842
87	40	NA	96	4.9	480	824	312	33	0.41	0.37	7.3	3	843
44	18	NA	24	2.3	143	670	0	0	0.24	0.27	3.6	Tr	844
51	31	NA	19	3.3	166	480	58	6	0.22	0.40	3.7	3	845
79	56	NA	102	6.2	263	973	207	37	0.28	0.70	4.2	0	846
135	35	NA	69	1.4	188	965	94	27	0.00	0.02	2.0	0	847
2	13	NA	17	0.4	235	182	33	8	0.07	0.04	1.0	Tr	848
18	36	NA	272	1.3	172	816	559	92	0.19	0.37	1.5	1	849
14	31	NA	73	0.8	129	430	8	1	0.08	0.10	0.9	1	850
9	21	NA	117	0.6	110	336	382	74	0.18	0.16	2.5	1	851
21	21	NA	101	1.5	179	382	524	101	0.21	0.17	2.0	2	852
14	20	NA	65	0.9	153	267	282	55	0.13	0.23	3.0	2	853
51	33	NA	54	4.2	316	792	210	21	0.38	0.31	5.9	2	854
72	4	NA	37	1.1	447	209	935	96	0.11	0.13	5.9	17	855
98	5	NA	100	0.7	371	119	822	115	0.09	0.17	1.0	10	856
43	68	2.7	376	1.0	666	323	310	77	0.19	0.82	0.5	1	857
37	60	1.3	406	0.3	579	273	433	107	0.15	0.61	0.6	3	858
200	40	NA	84	3.0	184	1,446	120	36	0.21	0.90	0.0	0	859
36	51	NA	189	2.5	394	1,651	424	80	1.00	0.80	5.5	12	860
73	44	NA	41	2.8	330	845	413	50	0.41	0.41	6.0	6	861
49	55	NA	74	2.6	335	1,293	187	41	0.46	0.33	11.3	4	862
56	27	NA	221	2.4	474	802	855	147	0.15	0.44	3.2	2	863
87	41	NA	339	3.7	729	1,233	1,315	226	0.24	0.68	4.9	3	864
44	24	NA	192	2.3	416	762	588	77	0.10	0.36	2.5	4	865
74	30	NA	189	2.5	491	871	1,276	173	0.09	0.50	2.9	4	866
20	16	NA	212	0.8	326	401	879	109	0.07	0.29	1.0	2	867

Table 9. Nutritive Value of the Edible Part of Food

Food No.	Food Description	Measure of edible portion	Weight (g)	Water (%)	Calories (kcal)	Protein (g)	Total fat (g)	Fatty acids Saturated (g)	Fatty acids Mono-unsaturated (g)	Fatty acids Poly-unsaturated (g)
	Poultry and Poultry Products									
	Chicken									
	Fried in vegetable shortening, meat with skin									
	Batter dipped									
868	Breast, ½ breast (5.6 oz with bones)	½ breast	140	52	364	35	18	4.9	7.6	4.3
869	Drumstick (3.4 oz with bones)	1 drumstick	72	53	193	16	11	3.0	4.6	2.7
870	Thigh	1 thigh	86	52	238	19	14	3.8	5.8	3.4
871	Wing	1 wing	49	46	159	10	11	2.9	4.4	2.5
	Flour coated									
872	Breast, ½ breast (4.2 oz with bones)	½ breast	98	57	218	31	9	2.4	3.4	1.9
873	Drumstick (2.6 oz with bones)	1 drumstick	49	57	120	13	7	1.8	2.7	1.6
	Fried, meat only									
874	Dark meat	3 oz	85	56	203	25	10	2.7	3.7	2.4
875	Light meat	3 oz	85	60	163	28	5	1.3	1.7	1.1
	Roasted, meat only									
876	Breast, ½ breast (4.2 oz with bone and skin)	½ breast	86	65	142	27	3	0.9	1.1	0.7
877	Drumstick (2.9 oz with bone and skin)	1 drumstick	44	67	76	12	2	0.7	0.8	0.6
878	Thigh	1 thigh	52	63	109	13	6	1.6	2.2	1.3
879	Stewed, meat only, light and dark meat, chopped or diced	1 cup	140	56	332	43	17	4.3	5.7	4.0
880	Chicken giblets, simmered, chopped	1 cup	145	68	228	37	7	2.2	1.7	1.6
881	Chicken liver, simmered	1 liver	20	68	31	5	1	0.4	0.3	0.2
882	Chicken neck, meat only, simmered	1 neck	18	67	32	4	1	0.4	0.5	0.4
883	Duck, roasted, flesh only	½ duck	221	64	444	52	25	9.2	8.2	3.2
	Turkey									
	Roasted, meat only									
884	Dark meat	3 oz	85	63	159	24	6	2.1	1.4	1.8
885	Light meat	3 oz	85	66	133	25	3	0.9	0.5	0.7
886	Light and dark meat, chopped or diced	1 cup	140	65	238	41	7	2.3	1.4	2.0
	Ground, cooked									
887	Patty, from 4 oz raw	1 patty	82	59	193	22	11	2.8	4.0	2.6
888	Crumbled	1 cup	127	59	298	35	17	4.3	6.2	4.1
889	Turkey giblets, simmered, chopped	1 cup	145	65	242	39	7	2.2	1.7	1.7
890	Turkey neck, meat only, simmered	1 neck	152	65	274	41	11	3.7	2.5	3.3
	Poultry food products									
	Chicken									
891	Canned, boneless	5 oz	142	69	234	31	11	3.1	4.5	2.5
892	Frankfurter (10 per 1 lb pkg)	1 frank	45	58	116	6	9	2.5	3.8	1.8
893	Roll, light meat (6 slices per 6-oz pkg)	2 slices	57	69	90	11	4	1.1	1.7	0.9

Choles-terol (mg)	Carbo-hydrate (g)	Total dietary fiber (g)	Calcium (mg)	Iron (mg)	Potas-sium (mg)	Sodium (mg)	Vitamin A		Thiamin (mg)	Ribo-flavin (mg)	Niacin (mg)	Ascor-bic acid (mg)	Food No.
							(IU)	(RE)					
119	13	0.4	28	1.8	281	385	94	28	0.16	0.20	14.7	0	868
62	6	0.2	12	1.0	134	194	62	19	0.08	0.15	3.7	0	869
80	8	0.3	15	1.2	165	248	82	25	0.10	0.20	4.9	0	870
39	5	0.1	10	0.6	68	157	55	17	0.05	0.07	2.6	0	871
87	2	0.1	16	1.2	254	74	49	15	0.08	0.13	13.5	0	872
44	1	Tr	6	0.7	112	44	41	12	0.04	0.11	3.0	0	873
82	2	0.0	15	1.3	215	82	67	20	0.08	0.21	6.0	0	874
77	Tr	0.0	14	1.0	224	69	26	8	0.06	0.11	11.4	0	875
73	0	0.0	13	0.9	220	64	18	5	0.06	0.10	11.8	0	876
41	0	0.0	5	0.6	108	42	26	8	0.03	0.10	2.7	0	877
49	0	0.0	6	0.7	124	46	34	10	0.04	0.12	3.4	0	878
116	0	0.0	18	2.0	283	109	157	46	0.16	0.39	9.0	0	879
570	1	0.0	17	9.3	229	84	10,775	3,232	0.13	1.38	5.9	12	880
126	Tr	0.0	3	1.7	28	10	3,275	983	0.03	0.35	0.9	3	881
14	0	0.0	8	0.5	25	12	22	6	0.01	0.05	0.7	0	882
197	0	0.0	27	6.0	557	144	170	51	0.57	1.04	11.3	0	883
72	0	0.0	27	2.0	247	67	0	0	0.05	0.21	3.1	0	884
59	0	0.0	16	1.1	259	54	0	0	0.05	0.11	5.8	0	885
106	0	0.0	35	2.5	417	98	0	0	0.09	0.25	7.6	0	886
84	0	0.0	21	1.6	221	88	0	0	0.04	0.14	4.0	0	887
130	0	0.0	32	2.5	343	136	0	0	0.07	0.21	6.1	0	888
606	3	0.0	19	9.7	290	86	8,752	2,603	0.07	1.31	6.5	2	889
185	0	0.0	56	3.5	226	85	0	0	0.05	0.29	2.6	0	890
88	0	0.0	20	2.2	196	714	166	48	0.02	0.18	9.0	3	891
45	3	0.0	43	0.9	38	617	59	17	0.03	0.05	1.4	0	892
28	1	0.0	24	0.5	129	331	46	14	0.04	0.07	3.0	0	893

Table 9. Nutritive Value of the Edible Part of Food

Food No.	Food Description	Measure of edible portion	Weight (g)	Water (%)	Calories (kcal)	Protein (g)	Total fat (g)	Fatty acids Saturated (g)	Mono-unsaturated (g)	Poly-unsaturated (g)
	Poultry and Poultry Products (continued)									
	Poultry food products (continued)									
	Turkey									
894	Gravy and turkey, frozen	5-oz package	142	85	95	8	4	1.2	1.4	0.7
895	Patties, breaded or battered, fried (2.25 oz)	1 patty	64	50	181	9	12	3.0	4.8	3.0
896	Roast, boneless, frozen, seasoned, light and dark meat, cooked	3 oz	85	68	132	18	5	1.6	1.0	1.4
	Soups, Sauces, and Gravies									
	Soups									
	Canned, condensed									
	Prepared with equal volume of whole milk									
897	Clam chowder, New England	1 cup	248	85	164	9	7	3.0	2.3	1.1
898	Cream of chicken	1 cup	248	85	191	7	11	4.6	4.5	1.6
899	Cream of mushroom	1 cup	248	85	203	6	14	5.1	3.0	4.6
900	Tomato	1 cup	248	85	161	6	6	2.9	1.6	1.1
	Prepared with equal volume of water									
901	Bean with pork	1 cup	253	84	172	8	6	1.5	2.2	1.8
902	Beef broth, bouillon, consomme	1 cup	241	96	29	5	0	0.0	0.0	0.0
903	Beef noodle	1 cup	244	92	83	5	3	1.1	1.2	0.5
904	Chicken noodle	1 cup	241	92	75	4	2	0.7	1.1	0.6
905	Chicken and rice	1 cup	241	94	60	4	2	0.5	0.9	0.4
906	Clam chowder, Manhattan	1 cup	244	92	78	2	2	0.4	0.4	1.3
907	Cream of chicken	1 cup	244	91	117	3	7	2.1	3.3	1.5
908	Cream of mushroom	1 cup	244	90	129	2	9	2.4	1.7	4.2
909	Minestrone	1 cup	241	91	82	4	3	0.6	0.7	1.1
910	Pea, green	1 cup	250	83	165	9	3	1.4	1.0	0.4
911	Tomato	1 cup	244	90	85	2	2	0.4	0.4	1.0
912	Vegetable beef	1 cup	244	92	78	6	2	0.9	0.8	0.1
913	Vegetarian vegetable	1 cup	241	92	72	2	2	0.3	0.8	0.7
	Canned, ready to serve, chunky									
914	Bean with ham	1 cup	243	79	231	13	9	3.3	3.8	0.9
915	Chicken noodle	1 cup	240	84	175	13	6	1.4	2.7	1.5
916	Chicken and vegetable	1 cup	240	83	166	12	5	1.4	2.2	1.0
917	Vegetable	1 cup	240	88	122	4	4	0.6	1.6	1.4
	Canned, ready to serve, low fat, reduced sodium									
918	Chicken broth	1 cup	240	97	17	3	0	0.0	0.0	0.0
919	Chicken noodle	1 cup	237	92	76	6	2	0.4	0.6	0.4
920	Chicken and rice	1 cup	241	88	116	7	3	0.9	1.3	0.7
921	Chicken and rice with vegetables	1 cup	239	91	88	6	1	0.4	0.5	0.5
922	Clam chowder, New England	1 cup	244	89	117	5	2	0.5	0.7	0.4
923	Lentil	1 cup	242	88	126	8	2	0.3	0.8	0.2
924	Minestrone	1 cup	241	87	123	5	3	0.4	0.9	1.0
925	Vegetable	1 cup	238	91	81	4	1	0.3	0.4	0.3

Choles-terol (mg)	Carbo-hydrate (g)	Total dietary fiber (g)	Calcium (mg)	Iron (mg)	Potas-sium (mg)	Sodium (mg)	Vitamin A (IU)	Vitamin A (RE)	Thiamin (mg)	Ribo-flavin (mg)	Niacin (mg)	Ascor-bic acid (mg)	Food No.
26	7	0.0	20	1.3	87	787	60	18	0.03	0.18	2.6	0	894
40	10	0.3	9	1.4	176	512	24	7	0.06	0.12	1.5	0	895
45	3	0.0	4	1.4	253	578	0	0	0.04	0.14	5.3	0	896
22	17	1.5	186	1.5	300	992	164	40	0.07	0.24	1.0	3	897
27	15	0.2	181	0.7	273	1,047	714	94	0.07	0.26	0.9	1	898
20	15	0.5	179	0.6	270	918	154	37	0.08	0.28	0.9	2	899
17	22	2.7	159	1.8	449	744	848	109	0.13	0.25	1.5	68	900
3	23	8.6	81	2.0	402	951	888	89	0.09	0.03	0.6	2	901
0	2	0.0	10	0.5	154	636	0	0	0.02	0.03	0.7	1	902
5	9	0.7	15	1.1	100	952	630	63	0.07	0.06	1.1	Tr	903
7	9	0.7	17	0.8	55	1,106	711	72	0.05	0.06	1.4	Tr	904
7	7	0.7	17	0.7	101	815	660	65	0.02	0.02	1.1	Tr	905
2	12	1.5	27	1.6	188	578	964	98	0.03	0.04	0.8	4	906
10	9	0.2	34	0.6	88	986	561	56	0.03	0.06	0.8	Tr	907
2	9	0.5	46	0.5	100	881	0	0	0.05	0.09	0.7	1	908
2	11	1.0	34	0.9	313	911	2,338	234	0.05	0.04	0.9	1	909
0	27	2.8	28	2.0	190	918	203	20	0.11	0.07	1.2	2	910
0	17	0.5	12	1.8	264	695	688	68	0.09	0.05	1.4	66	911
5	10	0.5	17	1.1	173	791	1,891	190	0.04	0.05	1.0	2	912
0	12	0.5	22	1.1	210	822	3,005	301	0.05	0.05	0.9	1	913
22	27	11.2	78	3.2	425	972	3,951	396	0.15	0.15	1.7	4	914
19	17	3.8	24	1.4	108	850	1,222	122	0.07	0.17	4.3	0	915
17	19	NA	26	1.5	367	1,068	5,990	600	0.04	0.17	3.3	6	916
0	19	1.2	55	1.6	396	1,010	5,878	588	0.07	0.06	1.2	6	917
0	1	0.0	19	0.6	204	554	0	0	Tr	0.03	1.6	1	918
19	9	1.2	19	1.1	209	460	920	95	0.11	0.11	3.4	1	919
14	14	0.7	22	1.0	422	482	2,010	202	0.05	0.13	5.0	2	920
17	12	0.7	24	1.2	275	459	1,644	165	0.12	0.07	2.6	1	921
5	20	1.2	17	0.9	283	529	244	59	0.05	0.09	0.9	5	922
0	20	5.6	41	2.7	336	443	951	94	0.11	0.09	0.7	1	923
0	20	1.2	39	1.7	306	470	1,357	135	0.15	0.08	1.0	1	924
5	13	1.4	31	1.5	290	466	3,196	319	0.08	0.07	1.8	1	925

Table 9. Nutritive Value of the Edible Part of Food

Food No.	Food Description	Measure of edible portion	Weight (g)	Water (%)	Calories (kcal)	Protein (g)	Total fat (g)	Fatty acids Saturated (g)	Mono-unsaturated (g)	Poly-unsaturated (g)
	Soups, Sauces, and Gravies (continued)									
	Soups (continued)									
	Dehydrated									
	Unprepared									
926	Beef bouillon	1 packet	6	3	14	1	1	0.3	0.2	Tr
927	Onion	1 packet	39	4	115	5	2	0.5	1.4	0.3
	Prepared with water									
928	Chicken noodle	1 cup	252	94	58	2	1	0.3	0.5	0.4
929	Onion	1 cup	246	96	27	1	1	0.1	0.3	0.1
	Home prepared, stock									
930	Beef	1 cup	240	96	31	5	Tr	0.1	0.1	Tr
931	Chicken	1 cup	240	92	86	6	3	0.8	1.4	0.5
932	Fish	1 cup	233	97	40	5	2	0.5	0.5	0.3
	Sauces									
	Home recipe									
933	Cheese	1 cup	243	67	479	25	36	19.5	11.5	3.4
934	White, medium, made with whole milk	1 cup	250	75	368	10	27	7.1	11.1	7.2
	Ready to serve									
935	Barbecue	1 tbsp	16	81	12	Tr	Tr	Tr	0.1	0.1
936	Cheese	¼ cup	63	71	110	4	8	3.8	2.4	1.6
937	Hoisin	1 tbsp	16	44	35	1	1	0.1	0.2	0.3
938	Nacho cheese	¼ cup	63	70	119	5	10	4.2	3.1	2.1
939	Pepper or hot	1 tsp	5	90	1	Tr	Tr	Tr	Tr	Tr
940	Salsa	1 tbsp	16	90	4	Tr	Tr	Tr	Tr	Tr
941	Soy	1 tbsp	16	69	9	1	Tr	Tr	Tr	Tr
942	Spaghetti/marinara/pasta	1 cup	250	87	143	4	5	0.7	2.2	1.8
943	Teriyaki	1 tbsp	18	68	15	1	0	0.0	0.0	0.0
944	Tomato chili	¼ cup	68	68	71	2	Tr	Tr	Tr	0.1
945	Worcestershire	1 tbsp	17	70	11	0	0	0.0	0.0	0.0
	Gravies, canned									
946	Beef	¼ cup	58	87	31	2	1	0.7	0.6	Tr
947	Chicken	¼ cup	60	85	47	1	3	0.8	1.5	0.9
948	Country sausage	¼ cup	62	75	96	3	8	2.0	2.9	2.2
949	Mushroom	¼ cup	60	89	30	1	2	0.2	0.7	0.6
950	Turkey	¼ cup	60	89	31	2	1	0.4	0.5	0.3
	Sugars and Sweets									
	Candy									
951	BUTTERFINGER (NESTLE)	1 fun size bar	7	2	34	1	1	0.7	0.4	0.2
	Caramel									
952	Plain	1 piece	10	9	39	Tr	1	0.7	0.1	Tr
953	Chocolate flavored roll	1 piece	7	7	25	Tr	Tr	Tr	0.1	0.1
954	Carob	1 oz	28	2	153	2	9	8.2	0.1	0.1
	Chocolate, milk									
955	Plain	1 bar (1.55 oz)	44	1	226	3	14	8.1	4.4	0.5
956	With almonds	1 bar (1.45 oz)	41	2	216	4	14	7.0	5.5	0.9
957	With peanuts, MR. GOODBAR (HERSHEY)	1 bar (1.75 oz)	49	1	267	5	17	7.3	5.7	2.4
958	With rice cereal, NESTLE CRUNCH	1 bar (1.55 oz)	44	1	230	3	12	6.7	3.8	0.4
	Chocolate chips									
959	Milk	1 cup	168	1	862	12	52	31.0	16.7	1.8
960	Semisweet	1 cup	168	1	805	7	50	29.8	16.7	1.6
961	White	1 cup	170	1	916	10	55	33.0	15.5	1.7
962	Chocolate coated peanuts	10 pieces	40	2	208	5	13	5.8	5.2	1.7
963	Chocolate coated raisins	10 pieces	10	11	39	Tr	1	0.9	0.5	0.1
964	Fruit leather, pieces	1 oz	28	12	97	Tr	2	0.3	0.9	0.8

Choles-terol (mg)	Carbo-hydrate (g)	Total dietary fiber (g)	Calcium (mg)	Iron (mg)	Potas-sium (mg)	Sodium (mg)	Vitamin A		Thiamin (mg)	Ribo-flavin (mg)	Niacin (mg)	Ascor-bic acid (mg)	Food No.
							(IU)	(RE)					
1	1	0.0	4	0.1	27	1,019	3	Tr	Tr	0.01	0.3	0	926
2	21	4.1	55	0.6	260	3,493	8	1	0.11	0.24	2.0	1	927
10	9	0.3	5	0.5	33	578	15	5	0.20	0.08	1.1	0	928
0	5	1.0	12	0.1	64	849	2	0	0.03	0.06	0.5	Tr	929
0	3	0.0	19	0.6	444	475	0	0	0.08	0.22	2.1	0	930
7	8	0.0	7	0.5	252	343	0	0	0.08	0.20	3.8	Tr	931
2	0	0.0	7	Tr	336	363	0	0	0.08	0.18	2.8	Tr	932
92	13	0.2	756	0.9	345	1,198	1,473	389	0.11	0.59	0.5	1	933
18	23	0.5	295	0.8	390	885	1,383	138	0.17	0.46	1.0	2	934
0	2	0.2	3	0.1	28	130	139	14	Tr	Tr	0.1	1	935
18	4	0.3	116	0.1	19	522	199	40	Tr	0.07	Tr	Tr	936
Tr	7	0.4	5	0.2	19	258	2	Tr	Tr	0.03	0.2	Tr	937
20	3	0.5	118	0.2	20	492	128	32	Tr	0.08	Tr	Tr	938
0	Tr	0.1	Tr	Tr	7	124	14	1	Tr	Tr	Tr	4	939
0	1	0.3	5	0.2	34	69	96	10	0.01	0.01	0.1	2	940
0	1	0.1	3	0.3	64	871	0	0	0.01	0.03	0.4	0	941
0	21	4.0	55	1.8	738	1,030	938	95	0.14	0.10	2.7	20	942
0	3	Tr	5	0.3	41	690	0	0	0.01	0.01	0.2	0	943
0	17	4.0	14	0.5	252	910	462	46	0.06	0.05	1.1	11	944
0	3	0.0	18	0.9	136	167	18	2	0.01	0.02	0.1	2	945
2	3	0.2	3	0.4	47	325	0	0	0.02	0.02	0.4	0	946
1	3	0.2	12	0.3	65	346	221	67	0.01	0.03	0.3	0	947
13	4	0.4	4	0.3	48	236	0	0	0.10	0.04	0.7	Tr	948
0	3	0.2	4	0.4	64	342	0	0	0.02	0.04	0.4	0	949
1	3	0.2	2	0.4	65	346	0	0	0.01	0.05	0.8	0	950
Tr	5	0.2	2	0.1	27	14	0	0	0.01	Tr	0.2	0	951
1	8	0.1	14	Tr	22	25	3	1	Tr	0.02	Tr	Tr	952
0	6	Tr	2	Tr	7	6	1	Tr	Tr	0.01	Tr	Tr	953
1	16	1.1	86	0.4	179	30	7	2	0.03	0.05	0.3	Tr	954
10	26	1.5	84	0.6	169	36	81	24	0.03	0.13	0.1	Tr	955
8	22	2.5	92	0.7	182	30	30	6	0.02	0.18	0.3	Tr	956
4	25	1.7	53	0.6	219	73	70	18	0.08	0.12	1.6	Tr	957
6	29	1.1	74	0.2	151	59	30	9	0.15	0.25	1.7	Tr	958
37	99	5.7	321	2.3	647	138	311	92	0.13	0.51	0.5	1	959
0	106	9.9	54	5.3	613	18	35	3	0.09	0.15	0.7	0	960
36	101	0.0	338	0.4	486	153	60	2	0.11	0.48	1.3	1	961
4	20	1.9	42	0.5	201	16	0	0	0.05	0.07	1.7	0	962
Tr	7	0.4	9	0.2	51	4	4	1	0.01	0.02	Tr	Tr	963
0	22	1.0	5	0.2	46	114	33	3	0.01	0.03	Tr	16	964

Table 9. Nutritive Value of the Edible Part of Food

Food No.	Food Description	Measure of edible portion	Weight (g)	Water (%)	Calories (kcal)	Protein (g)	Total fat (g)	Fatty acids		
								Saturated (g)	Mono-unsaturated (g)	Poly-unsaturated (g)

Sugars and Sweets (continued)

Food No.	Food Description	Measure of edible portion	Weight (g)	Water (%)	Calories (kcal)	Protein (g)	Total fat (g)	Saturated (g)	Mono-unsaturated (g)	Poly-unsaturated (g)
	Candy (continued)									
965	Fruit leather, rolls	1 large	21	11	74	Tr	1	0.1	0.3	0.1
966		1 small	14	11	49	Tr	Tr	0.1	0.2	0.1
	Fudge, prepared from recipe									
	Chocolate									
967	Plain	1 piece	17	10	65	Tr	1	0.9	0.4	0.1
968	With nuts	1 piece	19	7	81	1	3	1.1	0.8	1.0
	Vanilla									
969	Plain	1 piece	16	11	59	Tr	1	0.5	0.2	Tr
970	With nuts	1 piece	15	8	62	Tr	2	0.6	0.5	0.8
	Gumdrops/gummy candies									
971	Gumdrops (¾" dia)	1 cup	182	1	703	0	0	0.0	0.0	0.0
972		1 medium	4	1	16	0	0	0.0	0.0	0.0
973	Gummy bears	10 bears	22	1	85	0	0	0.0	0.0	0.0
974	Gummy worms	10 worms	74	1	286	0	0	0.0	0.0	0.0
975	Hard candy	1 piece	6	1	24	0	Tr	0.0	0.0	0.0
976		1 small piece	3	1	12	0	Tr	0.0	0.0	0.0
977	Jelly beans	10 large	28	6	104	0	Tr	Tr	0.1	Tr
978		10 small	11	6	40	0	Tr	Tr	Tr	Tr
979	KIT KAT (HERSHEY)	1 bar (1.5 oz)	42	2	216	3	11	6.8	3.1	0.3
	Marshmallows									
980	Miniature	1 cup	50	16	159	1	Tr	Tr	Tr	Tr
981	Regular	1 regular	7	16	23	Tr	Tr	Tr	Tr	Tr
	M&M's (M&M MARS)									
982	Peanut	¼ cup	43	2	222	4	11	4.4	4.7	1.8
983		10 pieces	20	2	103	2	5	2.1	2.2	0.8
984	Plain	¼ cup	52	2	256	2	11	6.8	3.6	0.3
985		10 pieces	7	2	34	Tr	1	0.9	0.5	Tr
986	MILKY WAY (M&M MARS)	1 fun size bar	18	6	76	1	3	1.4	1.1	0.1
987		1 bar (2.15 oz)	61	6	258	3	10	4.8	3.7	0.4
988	REESE'S Peanut butter cup (HERSHEY)	1 miniature cup	7	2	38	1	2	0.8	0.9	0.4
989		1 package (contains 2)	45	2	243	5	14	5.0	5.9	2.5
990	SNICKERS bar (M&M MARS)	1 fun size bar	15	5	72	1	4	1.3	1.6	0.7
991		1 king size bar (4 oz)	113	5	541	9	28	10.2	11.8	5.6
992		1 bar (2 oz)	57	5	273	5	14	5.1	6.0	2.8
993	SPECIAL DARK sweet chocolate (HERSHEY)	1 miniature	8	1	46	Tr	3	1.7	0.9	0.1
994	STARBURST fruit chews (M&M MARS)	1 piece	5	7	20	Tr	Tr	0.1	0.2	0.2
995		1 package (2.07 oz)	59	7	234	Tr	5	0.7	2.1	1.8
	Frosting, ready to eat									
996	Chocolate	1/12 package	38	17	151	Tr	7	2.1	3.4	0.8
997	Vanilla	1/12 package	38	13	159	Tr	6	1.9	3.3	0.9
	Frozen desserts (nondairy)									
998	Fruit and juice bar	1 bar (2.5 fl oz)	77	78	63	1	Tr	0.0	0.0	Tr
999	Ice pop	1 bar (2 fl oz)	59	80	42	0	0	0.0	0.0	0.0
1000	Italian ices	½ cup	116	86	61	Tr	Tr	0.0	0.0	0.0
1001	Fruit butter, apple	1 tbsp	17	56	29	Tr	0	0.0	0.0	0.0
	Gelatin dessert, prepared with gelatin dessert powder and water									
1002	Regular	½ cup	135	85	80	2	0	0.0	0.0	0.0
1003	Reduced calorie (with aspartame)	½ cup	117	98	8	1	0	0.0	0.0	0.0

Choles-terol (mg)	Carbo-hydrate (g)	Total dietary fiber (g)	Calcium (mg)	Iron (mg)	Potas-sium (mg)	Sodium (mg)	Vitamin A (IU)	Vitamin A (RE)	Thiamin (mg)	Ribo-flavin (mg)	Niacin (mg)	Ascor-bic acid (mg)	Food No.
0	18	0.8	7	0.2	62	13	24	3	0.01	Tr	Tr	1	965
0	12	0.5	4	0.1	41	9	16	2	0.01	Tr	Tr	1	966
2	14	0.1	7	0.1	18	11	32	8	Tr	0.01	Tr	Tr	967
3	14	0.2	10	0.1	30	11	38	9	0.01	0.02	Tr	Tr	968
3	13	0.0	6	Tr	8	11	33	8	Tr	0.01	Tr	Tr	969
2	11	0.1	7	0.1	17	9	30	7	0.01	0.01	Tr	Tr	970
0	180	0.0	5	0.7	9	80	0	0	0.00	Tr	Tr	0	971
0	4	0.0	Tr	Tr	Tr	2	0	0	0.00	Tr	Tr	0	972
0	22	0.0	1	0.1	1	10	0	0	0.00	Tr	Tr	0	973
0	73	0.0	2	0.3	4	33	0	0	0.00	Tr	Tr	0	974
0	6	0.0	Tr	Tr	Tr	2	0	0	Tr	Tr	Tr	0	975
0	3	0.0	Tr	Tr	Tr	1	0	0	Tr	Tr	Tr	0	976
0	26	0.0	1	0.3	10	7	0	0	0.00	0.00	0.0	0	977
0	10	0.0	Tr	0.1	4	3	0	0	0.00	0.00	0.0	0	978
3	27	0.8	69	0.4	122	32	68	20	0.07	0.23	1.1	Tr	979
0	41	0.1	2	0.1	3	24	1	0	Tr	Tr	Tr	0	980
0	6	Tr	Tr	Tr	Tr	3	Tr	0	Tr	Tr	Tr	0	981
4	26	1.5	43	0.5	149	21	40	10	0.04	0.07	1.6	Tr	982
2	12	0.7	20	0.2	69	10	19	5	0.02	0.03	0.7	Tr	983
7	37	1.3	55	0.6	138	32	106	28	0.03	0.11	0.1	Tr	984
1	5	0.2	7	0.1	19	4	14	4	Tr	0.01	Tr	Tr	985
3	13	0.3	23	0.1	43	43	19	6	0.01	0.04	0.1	Tr	986
9	44	1.0	79	0.5	147	146	66	20	0.02	0.14	0.2	1	987
Tr	4	0.2	5	0.1	25	22	5	1	0.02	0.01	0.3	Tr	988
2	25	1.4	35	0.5	158	143	33	9	0.11	0.08	2.1	Tr	989
2	9	0.4	14	0.1	49	40	23	6	0.01	0.02	0.6	Tr	990
15	67	2.8	106	0.9	366	301	172	44	0.11	0.17	4.7	1	991
7	34	1.4	54	0.4	185	152	87	22	0.06	0.09	2.4	Tr	992
Tr	5	0.4	2	0.2	25	1	3	Tr	Tr	0.01	Tr	0	993
0	4	0.0	Tr	Tr	Tr	3	0	0	Tr	Tr	Tr	3	994
0	50	0.0	2	0.1	1	33	0	0	Tr	Tr	Tr	31	995
0	24	0.2	3	0.5	74	70	249	75	Tr	0.01	Tr	0	996
0	26	Tr	1	Tr	14	34	283	86	0.00	Tr	Tr	0	997
0	16	0.0	4	0.1	41	3	22	2	0.01	0.01	0.1	7	998
0	11	0.0	0	0.0	2	7	0	0	0.00	0.00	0.0	0	999
0	16	0.0	1	0.1	7	5	194	0	0.01	0.01	0.8	1	1000
0	7	0.3	2	0.1	15	1	20	2	Tr	Tr	Tr	Tr	1001
0	19	0.0	3	Tr	1	57	0	0	0.00	Tr	Tr	0	1002
0	1	0.0	2	Tr	0	56	0	0	0.00	Tr	Tr	0	1003

Table 9. Nutritive Value of the Edible Part of Food

Food No.	Food Description	Measure of edible portion	Weight (g)	Water (%)	Calories (kcal)	Protein (g)	Total fat (g)	Fatty acids Saturated (g)	Mono-unsaturated (g)	Poly-unsaturated (g)
	Sugars and Sweets (continued)									
1004	Honey, strained or extracted	1 tbsp	21	17	64	Tr	0	0.0	0.0	0.0
1005		1 cup	339	17	1,031	1	0	0.0	0.0	0.0
1006	Jams and preserves	1 tbsp	20	30	56	Tr	Tr	Tr	Tr	0.0
1007		1 packet (0.5 oz)	14	30	39	Tr	Tr	Tr	Tr	0.0
1008	Jellies	1 tbsp	19	29	54	Tr	Tr	Tr	Tr	Tr
1009		1 packet (0.5 oz)	14	29	40	Tr	Tr	Tr	Tr	Tr
	Puddings									
	Prepared with dry mix and 2% milk									
	Chocolate									
1010	Instant	½ cup	147	75	150	5	3	1.6	0.9	0.2
1011	Regular (cooked)	½ cup	142	74	151	5	3	1.8	0.8	0.1
	Vanilla									
1012	Instant	½ cup	142	75	148	4	2	1.4	0.7	0.1
1013	Regular (cooked)	½ cup	140	76	141	4	2	1.5	0.7	0.1
	Ready to eat									
	Regular									
1014	Chocolate	4 oz	113	69	150	3	5	0.8	1.9	1.6
1015	Rice	4 oz	113	68	184	2	8	1.3	3.6	3.2
1016	Tapioca	4 oz	113	74	134	2	4	0.7	1.8	1.5
1017	Vanilla	4 oz	113	71	147	3	4	0.6	1.7	1.5
	Fat free									
1018	Chocolate	4 oz	113	76	107	3	Tr	0.3	0.1	Tr
1019	Tapioca	4 oz	113	77	98	2	Tr	0.1	Tr	Tr
1020	Vanilla	4 oz	113	76	105	2	Tr	0.1	Tr	Tr
	Sugar									
	Brown									
1021	Packed	1 cup	220	2	827	0	0	0.0	0.0	0.0
1022	Unpacked	1 cup	145	2	545	0	0	0.0	0.0	0.0
1023		1 tbsp	9	2	34	0	0	0.0	0.0	0.0
	White									
1024	Granulated	1 packet	6	0	23	0	0	0.0	0.0	0.0
1025		1 tsp	4	0	16	0	0	0.0	0.0	0.0
1026		1 cup	200	0	774	0	0	0.0	0.0	0.0
1027	Powdered, unsifted	1 tbsp	8	Tr	31	0	Tr	Tr	Tr	Tr
1028		1 cup	120	Tr	467	0	Tr	Tr	Tr	0.1
	Syrup									
	Chocolate flavored syrup or topping									
1029	Thin type	1 tbsp	19	31	53	Tr	Tr	0.1	0.1	Tr
1030	Fudge type	1 tbsp	19	22	67	1	2	0.8	0.7	0.1
1031	Corn, light	1 tbsp	20	23	56	0	0	0.0	0.0	0.0
1032	Maple	1 tbsp	20	32	52	0	Tr	Tr	Tr	Tr
1033	Molasses, blackstrap	1 tbsp	20	29	47	0	0	0.0	0.0	0.0
1034		1 cup	328	29	771	0	0	0.0	0.0	0.0
	Table blend, pancake									
1035	Regular	1 tbsp	20	24	57	0	0	0.0	0.0	0.0
1036	Reduced calorie	1 tbsp	15	55	25	0	0	0.0	0.0	0.0

Choles-terol (mg)	Carbo-hydrate (g)	Total dietary fiber (g)	Calcium (mg)	Iron (mg)	Potas-sium (mg)	Sodium (mg)	Vitamin A (IU)	Vitamin A (RE)	Thiamin (mg)	Ribo-flavin (mg)	Niacin (mg)	Ascor-bic acid (mg)	Food No.
0	17	Tr	1	0.1	11	1	0	0	0.00	0.01	Tr	Tr	1004
0	279	0.7	20	1.4	176	14	0	0	0.00	0.13	0.4	2	1005
0	14	0.2	4	0.1	15	6	2	Tr	0.00	Tr	Tr	2	1006
0	10	0.2	3	0.1	11	4	2	Tr	0.00	Tr	Tr	1	1007
0	13	0.2	2	Tr	12	5	3	Tr	Tr	Tr	Tr	Tr	1008
0	10	0.1	1	Tr	9	4	2	Tr	Tr	Tr	Tr	Tr	1009
9	28	0.6	153	0.4	247	417	253	56	0.05	0.21	0.1	1	1010
10	28	0.4	160	0.5	240	149	253	68	0.05	0.21	0.2	1	1011
9	28	0.0	146	0.1	185	406	241	64	0.05	0.20	0.1	1	1012
10	26	0.0	153	0.1	193	224	252	70	0.04	0.20	0.1	1	1013
3	26	1.1	102	0.6	203	146	41	12	0.03	0.18	0.4	2	1014
1	25	0.1	59	0.3	68	96	129	40	0.02	0.08	0.2	1	1015
1	22	0.1	95	0.3	110	180	0	0	0.02	0.11	0.4	1	1016
8	25	0.1	99	0.1	128	153	24	7	0.02	0.16	0.3	0	1017
2	23	0.9	89	0.6	235	192	174	52	0.02	0.12	0.1	Tr	1018
1	23	0.1	76	0.2	99	251	121	36	0.02	0.09	0.1	Tr	1019
1	24	0.1	86	Tr	123	241	174	52	0.02	0.10	0.1	Tr	1020
0	214	0.0	187	4.2	761	86	0	0	0.02	0.02	0.2	0	1021
0	141	0.0	123	2.8	502	57	0	0	0.01	0.01	0.1	0	1022
0	9	0.0	8	0.2	31	4	0	0	Tr	Tr	Tr	0	1023
0	6	0.0	Tr	Tr	Tr	Tr	0	0	0.00	Tr	0.0	0	1024
0	4	0.0	Tr	Tr	Tr	Tr	0	0	0.00	Tr	0.0	0	1025
0	200	0.0	2	0.1	4	2	0	0	0.00	0.04	0.0	0	1026
0	8	0.0	Tr	Tr	Tr	Tr	0	0	0.00	0.00	0.0	0	1027
0	119	0.0	1	0.1	2	1	0	0	0.00	0.00	0.0	0	1028
0	12	0.3	3	0.4	43	14	6	1	Tr	0.01	0.1	Tr	1029
Tr	12	0.5	15	0.2	69	66	3	1	0.01	0.04	0.1	Tr	1030
0	15	0.0	1	Tr	1	24	0	0	Tr	Tr	Tr	0	1031
0	13	0.0	13	0.2	41	2	0	0	Tr	Tr	Tr	0	1032
0	12	0.0	172	3.5	498	11	0	0	0.01	0.01	0.2	0	1033
0	199	0.0	2,821	57.4	8,174	180	0	0	0.11	0.17	3.5	0	1034
0	15	0.0	Tr	Tr	Tr	17	0	0	Tr	Tr	Tr	0	1035
0	7	0.0	Tr	Tr	Tr	30	0	0	Tr	Tr	Tr	0	1036

Table 9. Nutritive Value of the Edible Part of Food

Food No.	Food Description	Measure of edible portion	Weight (g)	Water (%)	Calories (kcal)	Protein (g)	Total fat (g)	Fatty acids Saturated (g)	Mono-unsaturated (g)	Poly-unsaturated (g)
	Vegetables and Vegetable Products									
1037	Alfalfa sprouts, raw	1 cup	33	91	10	1	Tr	Tr	Tr	0.1
1038	Artichokes, globe or French, cooked, drained	1 cup	168	84	84	6	Tr	0.1	Tr	0.1
1039		1 medium	120	84	60	4	Tr	Tr	Tr	0.1
	Asparagus, green Cooked, drained									
1040	From raw	1 cup	180	92	43	5	1	0.1	Tr	0.2
1041		4 spears	60	92	14	2	Tr	Tr	Tr	0.1
1042	From frozen	1 cup	180	91	50	5	1	0.2	Tr	0.3
1043		4 spears	60	91	17	2	Tr	0.1	Tr	0.1
1044	Canned, spears, about 5" long, drained	1 cup	242	94	46	5	2	0.4	0.1	0.7
1045		4 spears	72	94	14	2	Tr	0.1	Tr	0.2
1046	Bamboo shoots, canned, drained	1 cup	131	94	25	2	1	0.1	Tr	0.2
	Beans Lima, immature seeds, frozen, cooked, drained									
1047	Ford hooks	1 cup	170	74	170	10	1	0.1	Tr	0.3
1048	Baby limas	1 cup	180	72	189	12	1	0.1	Tr	0.3
	Snap, cut Cooked, drained From raw									
1049	Green	1 cup	125	89	44	2	Tr	0.1	Tr	0.2
1050	Yellow	1 cup	125	89	44	2	Tr	0.1	Tr	0.2
	From frozen									
1051	Green	1 cup	135	91	38	2	Tr	0.1	Tr	0.1
1052	Yellow	1 cup	135	91	38	2	Tr	0.1	Tr	0.1
	Canned, drained									
1053	Green	1 cup	135	93	27	2	Tr	Tr	Tr	0.1
1054	Yellow	1 cup	135	93	27	2	Tr	Tr	Tr	0.1
	Beans, dry. See Legumes. Bean sprouts (mung)									
1055	Raw	1 cup	104	90	31	3	Tr	Tr	Tr	0.1
1056	Cooked, drained	1 cup	124	93	26	3	Tr	Tr	Tr	Tr
	Beets Cooked, drained									
1057	Slices	1 cup	170	87	75	3	Tr	Tr	0.1	0.1
1058	Whole beet, 2" dia	1 beet	50	87	22	1	Tr	Tr	Tr	Tr
	Canned, drained									
1059	Slices	1 cup	170	91	53	2	Tr	Tr	Tr	0.1
1060	Whole beet	1 beet	24	91	7	Tr	Tr	Tr	Tr	Tr
1061	Beet greens, leaves and stems, cooked, drained, 1" pieces	1 cup	144	89	39	4	Tr	Tr	0.1	0.1
	Black eyed peas, immature seeds, cooked, drained									
1062	From raw	1 cup	165	75	160	5	1	0.2	0.1	0.3
1063	From frozen	1 cup	170	66	224	14	1	0.3	0.1	0.5
	Broccoli Raw									
1064	Chopped or diced	1 cup	88	91	25	3	Tr	Tr	Tr	0.1
1065	Spear, about 5" long	1 spear	31	91	9	1	Tr	Tr	Tr	0.1
1066	Flower cluster	1 floweret	11	91	3	Tr	Tr	Tr	Tr	Tr
	Cooked, drained From raw									
1067	Chopped	1 cup	156	91	44	5	1	0.1	Tr	0.3
1068	Spear, about 5" long	1 spear	37	91	10	1	Tr	Tr	Tr	0.1
1069	From frozen, chopped	1 cup	184	91	52	6	Tr	Tr	Tr	0.1

Choles-terol (mg)	Carbo-hydrate (g)	Total dietary fiber (g)	Calcium (mg)	Iron (mg)	Potas-sium (mg)	Sodium (mg)	Vitamin A (IU)	Vitamin A (RE)	Thiamin (mg)	Ribo-flavin (mg)	Niacin (mg)	Ascor-bic acid (mg)	Food No.
0	1	0.8	11	0.3	26	2	51	5	0.03	0.04	0.2	3	1037
0	19	9.1	76	2.2	595	160	297	30	0.11	0.11	1.7	17	1038
0	13	6.5	54	1.5	425	114	212	22	0.08	0.08	1.2	12	1039
0	8	2.9	36	1.3	288	20	970	97	0.22	0.23	1.9	19	1040
0	3	1.0	12	0.4	96	7	323	32	0.07	0.08	0.6	6	1041
0	9	2.9	41	1.2	392	7	1,472	148	0.12	0.19	1.9	44	1042
0	3	1.0	14	0.4	131	2	491	49	0.04	0.06	0.6	15	1043
0	6	3.9	39	4.4	416	695	1,285	128	0.15	0.24	2.3	45	1044
0	2	1.2	12	1.3	124	207	382	38	0.04	0.07	0.7	13	1045
0	4	1.8	10	0.4	105	9	10	1	0.03	0.03	0.2	1	1046
0	32	9.9	37	2.3	694	90	323	32	0.13	0.10	1.8	22	1047
0	35	10.8	50	3.5	740	52	301	31	0.13	0.10	1.4	10	1048
0	10	4.0	58	1.6	374	4	833	84	0.09	0.12	0.8	12	1049
0	10	4.1	58	1.6	374	4	101	10	0.09	0.12	0.8	12	1050
0	9	4.1	66	1.2	170	12	541	54	0.05	0.12	0.5	6	1051
0	9	4.1	66	1.2	170	12	151	15	0.05	0.12	0.5	6	1052
0	6	2.6	35	1.2	147	354	471	47	0.02	0.08	0.3	6	1053
0	6	1.8	35	1.2	147	339	142	15	0.02	0.08	0.3	6	1054
0	6	1.9	14	0.9	155	6	22	2	0.09	0.13	0.8	14	1055
0	5	1.5	15	0.8	125	12	17	1	0.06	0.13	1.0	14	1056
0	17	3.4	27	1.3	519	131	60	7	0.05	0.07	0.6	6	1057
0	5	1.0	8	0.4	153	39	18	2	0.01	0.02	0.2	2	1058
0	12	2.9	26	3.1	252	330	19	2	0.02	0.07	0.3	7	1059
0	2	0.4	4	0.4	36	47	3	Tr	Tr	0.01	Tr	1	1060
0	8	4.2	164	2.7	1,309	347	7,344	734	0.17	0.42	0.7	36	1061
0	34	8.3	211	1.8	690	7	1,305	130	0.17	0.24	2.3	4	1062
0	40	10.9	39	3.6	638	9	128	14	0.44	0.11	1.2	4	1063
0	5	2.6	42	0.8	286	24	1,357	136	0.06	0.10	0.6	82	1064
0	2	0.9	15	0.3	101	8	478	48	0.02	0.04	0.2	29	1065
0	1	0.3	5	0.1	36	3	330	33	0.01	0.01	0.1	10	1066
0	8	4.5	72	1.3	456	41	2,165	217	0.09	0.18	0.9	116	1067
0	2	1.1	17	0.3	108	10	514	51	0.02	0.04	0.2	28	1068
0	10	5.5	94	1.1	331	44	3,481	348	0.10	0.15	0.8	74	1069

Table 9. Nutritive Value of the Edible Part of Food

Food No.	Food Description	Measure of edible portion	Weight (g)	Water (%)	Calories (kcal)	Protein (g)	Total fat (g)	Saturated (g)	Mono-unsaturated (g)	Poly-unsaturated (g)
	Vegetables and Vegetable Products (continued)									
	Brussels sprouts, cooked, drained									
1070	From raw	1 cup	156	87	61	4	1	0.2	0.1	0.4
1071	From frozen	1 cup	155	87	65	6	1	0.1	Tr	0.3
	Cabbage, common varieties, shredded									
1072	Raw	1 cup	70	92	18	1	Tr	Tr	Tr	0.1
1073	Cooked, drained	1 cup	150	94	33	2	1	0.1	Tr	0.3
	Cabbage, Chinese, shredded, cooked, drained									
1074	Pak choi or bok choy	1 cup	170	96	20	3	Tr	Tr	Tr	0.1
1075	Pe tsai	1 cup	119	95	17	2	Tr	Tr	Tr	0.1
1076	Cabbage, red, raw, shredded	1 cup	70	92	19	1	Tr	Tr	Tr	0.1
1077	Cabbage, savoy, raw, shredded	1 cup	70	91	19	1	Tr	Tr	Tr	Tr
1078	Carrot juice, canned	1 cup	236	89	94	2	Tr	0.1	Tr	0.2
	Carrots									
	Raw									
1079	Whole, 7½" long	1 carrot	72	88	31	1	Tr	Tr	Tr	0.1
1080	Grated	1 cup	110	88	47	1	Tr	Tr	Tr	0.1
1081	Baby	1 medium	10	90	4	Tr	Tr	Tr	Tr	Tr
	Cooked, sliced, drained									
1082	From raw	1 cup	156	87	70	2	Tr	0.1	Tr	0.1
1083	From frozen	1 cup	146	90	53	2	Tr	Tr	Tr	0.1
1084	Canned, sliced, drained	1 cup	146	93	37	1	Tr	0.1	Tr	0.1
	Cauliflower									
1085	Raw	1 floweret	13	92	3	Tr	Tr	Tr	Tr	Tr
1086		1 cup	100	92	25	2	Tr	Tr	Tr	0.1
	Cooked, drained, 1" pieces									
1087	From raw	1 cup	124	93	29	2	1	0.1	Tr	0.3
1088		3 flowerets	54	93	12	1	Tr	Tr	Tr	0.1
1089	From frozen	1 cup	180	94	34	3	Tr	0.1	Tr	0.2
	Celery									
	Raw									
1090	Stalk, 7½ to 8" long	1 stalk	40	95	6	Tr	Tr	Tr	Tr	Tr
1091	Pieces, diced	1 cup	120	95	19	1	Tr	Tr	Tr	0.1
	Cooked, drained									
1092	Stalk, medium	1 stalk	38	94	7	Tr	Tr	Tr	Tr	Tr
1093	Pieces, diced	1 cup	150	94	27	1	Tr	0.1	Tr	0.1
1094	Chives, raw, chopped	1 tbsp	3	91	1	Tr	Tr	Tr	Tr	Tr
1095	Cilantro, raw	1 tsp	2	92	Tr	Tr	Tr	Tr	Tr	Tr
1096	Coleslaw, home prepared	1 cup	120	82	83	2	3	0.5	0.8	1.6
	Collards, cooked, drained, chopped									
1097	From raw	1 cup	190	92	49	4	1	0.1	Tr	0.3
1098	From frozen	1 cup	170	88	61	5	1	0.1	Tr	0.4
	Corn, sweet, yellow									
	Cooked, drained									
1099	From raw, kernels on cob	1 ear	77	70	83	3	1	0.2	0.3	0.5
	From frozen									
1100	Kernels on cob	1 ear	63	73	59	2	Tr	0.1	0.1	0.2
1101	Kernels	1 cup	164	77	131	5	1	0.1	0.2	0.3
	Canned									
1102	Cream style	1 cup	256	79	184	4	1	0.2	0.3	0.5
1103	Whole kernel, vacuum pack	1 cup	210	77	166	5	1	0.2	0.3	0.5
1104	Corn, sweet, white, cooked, drained	1 ear	77	70	83	3	1	0.2	0.3	0.5

*White varieties contain only a trace amount of vitamin A; other nutrients are the same.

Choles-terol (mg)	Carbo-hydrate (g)	Total dietary fiber (g)	Calcium (mg)	Iron (mg)	Potas-sium (mg)	Sodium (mg)	Vitamin A (IU)	Vitamin A (RE)	Thiamin (mg)	Ribo-flavin (mg)	Niacin (mg)	Ascor-bic acid (mg)	Food No.
0	14	4.1	56	1.9	495	33	1,122	112	0.17	0.12	0.9	97	1070
0	13	6.4	37	1.1	504	36	913	91	0.16	0.18	0.8	71	1071
0	4	1.6	33	0.4	172	13	93	9	0.04	0.03	0.2	23	1072
0	7	3.5	47	0.3	146	12	198	20	0.09	0.08	0.4	30	1073
0	3	2.7	158	1.8	631	58	4,366	437	0.05	0.11	0.7	44	1074
0	3	3.2	38	0.4	268	11	1,151	115	0.05	0.05	0.6	19	1075
0	4	1.4	36	0.3	144	8	28	3	0.04	0.02	0.2	40	1076
0	4	2.2	25	0.3	161	20	700	70	0.05	0.02	0.2	22	1077
0	22	1.9	57	1.1	689	68	25,833	2,584	0.22	0.13	0.9	20	1078
0	7	2.2	19	0.4	233	25	20,253	2,025	0.07	0.04	0.7	7	1079
0	11	3.3	30	0.6	355	39	30,942	3,094	0.11	0.06	1.0	10	1080
0	1	0.2	2	0.1	28	4	1,501	150	Tr	0.01	0.1	1	1081
0	16	5.1	48	1.0	354	103	38,304	3,830	0.05	0.09	0.8	4	1082
0	12	5.1	41	0.7	231	86	25,845	2,584	0.04	0.05	0.6	4	1083
0	8	2.2	37	0.9	261	353	20,110	2,010	0.03	0.04	0.8	4	1084
0	1	0.3	3	0.1	39	4	2	Tr	0.01	0.01	0.1	6	1085
0	5	2.5	22	0.4	303	30	19	2	0.06	0.06	0.5	46	1086
0	5	3.3	20	0.4	176	19	21	2	0.05	0.06	0.5	55	1087
0	2	1.5	9	0.2	77	8	9	1	0.02	0.03	0.2	24	1088
0	7	4.9	31	0.7	250	32	40	4	0.07	0.10	0.6	56	1089
0	1	0.7	16	0.2	115	35	54	5	0.02	0.02	0.1	3	1090
0	4	2.0	48	0.5	344	104	161	16	0.06	0.05	0.4	8	1091
0	2	0.6	16	0.2	108	35	50	5	0.02	0.02	0.1	2	1092
0	6	2.4	63	0.6	426	137	198	20	0.06	0.07	0.5	9	1093
0	Tr	0.1	3	Tr	9	Tr	131	13	Tr	Tr	Tr	2	1094
0	Tr	Tr	1	Tr	8	1	98	10	Tr	Tr	Tr	1	1095
10	15	1.8	54	0.7	217	28	762	98	0.08	0.07	0.3	39	1096
0	9	5.3	226	0.9	494	17	5,945	595	0.08	0.20	1.1	35	1097
0	12	4.8	357	1.9	427	85	10,168	1,017	0.08	0.20	1.1	45	1098
0	19	2.2	2	0.5	192	13	167	17	0.17	0.06	1.2	5	1099
0	14	1.8	2	0.4	158	3	133*	13*	0.11	0.04	1.0	3	1100
0	32	3.9	7	0.6	241	8	361*	36*	0.14	0.12	2.1	5	1101
0	46	3.1	8	1.0	343	730	248*	26*	0.06	0.14	2.5	12	1102
0	41	4.2	11	0.9	391	571	506*	50*	0.09	0.15	2.5	17	1103
0	19	2.1	2	0.5	192	13	0	0	0.17	0.06	1.2	5	1104

Table 9. Nutritive Value of the Edible Part of Food

Food No.	Food Description	Measure of edible portion	Weight (g)	Water (%)	Calories (kcal)	Protein (g)	Total fat (g)	Fatty acids Saturated (g)	Mono-unsaturated (g)	Poly-unsaturated (g)
	Vegetables and Vegetable Products (continued)									
	Cucumber									
	Peeled									
1105	Sliced	1 cup	119	96	14	1	Tr	Tr	Tr	0.1
1106	Whole, 8¼" long	1 large	280	96	34	2	Tr	0.1	Tr	0.2
	Unpeeled									
1107	Sliced	1 cup	104	96	14	1	Tr	Tr	Tr	0.1
1108	Whole, 8¼" long	1 large	301	96	39	2	Tr	0.1	Tr	0.2
1109	Dandelion greens, cooked, drained	1 cup	105	90	35	2	1	0.2	Tr	0.3
1110	Dill weed, raw	5 sprigs	1	86	Tr	Tr	Tr	Tr	Tr	Tr
1111	Eggplant, cooked, drained	1 cup	99	92	28	1	Tr	Tr	Tr	0.1
1112	Endive, curly (including escarole), raw, small pieces	1 cup	50	94	9	1	Tr	Tr	Tr	Tr
1113	Garlic, raw	1 clove	3	59	4	Tr	Tr	Tr	Tr	Tr
1114	Hearts of palm, canned	1 piece	33	90	9	1	Tr	Tr	Tr	0.1
1115	Jerusalem artichoke, raw, sliced	1 cup	150	78	114	3	Tr	0.0	Tr	Tr
	Kale, cooked, drained, chopped									
1116	From raw	1 cup	130	91	36	2	1	0.1	Tr	0.3
1117	From frozen	1 cup	130	91	39	4	1	0.1	Tr	0.3
1118	Kohlrabi, cooked, drained, slices	1 cup	165	90	48	3	Tr	Tr	Tr	0.1
1119	Leeks, bulb and lower leaf portion, chopped or diced, cooked, drained	1 cup	104	91	32	1	Tr	Tr	Tr	0.1
	Lettuce, raw									
	Butterhead, as Boston types									
1120	Leaf	1 medium leaf	8	96	1	Tr	Tr	Tr	Tr	Tr
1121	Head, 5" dia	1 head	163	96	21	2	Tr	Tr	Tr	0.2
	Crisphead, as iceberg									
1122	Leaf	1 medium	8	96	1	Tr	Tr	Tr	Tr	Tr
1123	Head, 6" dia	1 head	539	96	65	5	1	0.1	Tr	0.5
1124	Pieces, shredded or chopped	1 cup	55	96	7	1	Tr	Tr	Tr	0.1
	Looseleaf									
1125	Leaf	1 leaf	10	94	2	Tr	Tr	Tr	Tr	Tr
1126	Pieces, shredded	1 cup	56	94	10	1	Tr	Tr	Tr	0.1
	Romaine or cos									
1127	Innerleaf	1 leaf	10	95	1	Tr	Tr	Tr	Tr	Tr
1128	Pieces, shredded	1 cup	56	95	8	1	Tr	Tr	Tr	0.1
	Mushrooms									
1129	Raw, pieces or slices	1 cup	70	92	18	2	Tr	Tr	Tr	0.1
1130	Cooked, drained, pieces	1 cup	156	91	42	3	1	0.1	Tr	0.3
1131	Canned, drained, pieces	1 cup	156	91	37	3	Tr	0.1	Tr	0.2
	Mushrooms, shiitake									
1132	Cooked pieces	1 cup	145	83	80	2	Tr	0.1	0.1	Tr
1133	Dried	1 mushroom	4	10	11	Tr	Tr	Tr	Tr	Tr
1134	Mustard greens, cooked, drained	1 cup	140	94	21	3	Tr	Tr	0.2	0.1
	Okra, sliced, cooked, drained									
1135	From raw	1 cup	160	90	51	3	Tr	0.1	Tr	0.1
1136	From frozen	1 cup	184	91	52	4	1	0.1	0.1	0.1
	Onions									
	Raw									
1137	Chopped	1 cup	160	90	61	2	Tr	Tr	Tr	0.1
1138	Whole, medium, 2½" dia	1 whole	110	90	42	1	Tr	Tr	Tr	0.1
1139	Slice, ⅛" thick	1 slice	14	90	5	Tr	Tr	Tr	Tr	Tr

Choles-terol (mg)	Carbo-hydrate (g)	Total dietary fiber (g)	Calcium (mg)	Iron (mg)	Potas-sium (mg)	Sodium (mg)	Vitamin A (IU)	Vitamin A (RE)	Thiamin (mg)	Ribo-flavin (mg)	Niacin (mg)	Ascor-bic acid (mg)	Food No.
0	3	0.8	17	0.2	176	2	88	8	0.02	0.01	0.1	3	1105
0	7	2.0	39	0.4	414	6	207	20	0.06	0.03	0.3	8	1106
0	3	0.8	15	0.3	150	2	224	22	0.02	0.02	0.2	6	1107
0	8	2.4	42	0.8	433	6	647	63	0.07	0.07	0.7	16	1108
0	7	3.0	147	1.9	244	46	12,285	1,229	0.14	0.18	0.5	19	1109
0	Tr	Tr	2	0.1	7	1	77	8	Tr	Tr	Tr	1	1110
0	7	2.5	6	0.3	246	3	63	6	0.08	0.02	0.6	1	1111
0	2	1.6	26	0.4	157	11	1,025	103	0.04	0.04	0.2	3	1112
0	1	0.1	5	0.1	12	1	0	0	0.01	Tr	Tr	1	1113
0	2	0.8	19	1.0	58	141	0	0	Tr	0.02	0.1	3	1114
0	26	2.4	21	5.1	644	6	30	3	0.30	0.09	2.0	6	1115
0	7	2.6	94	1.2	296	30	9,620	962	0.07	0.09	0.7	53	1116
0	7	2.6	179	1.2	417	20	8,260	826	0.06	0.15	0.9	33	1117
0	11	1.8	41	0.7	561	35	58	7	0.07	0.03	0.6	89	1118
0	8	1.0	31	1.1	90	10	48	5	0.03	0.02	0.2	4	1119
0	Tr	0.1	2	Tr	19	Tr	73	7	Tr	Tr	Tr	1	1120
0	4	1.6	52	0.5	419	8	1,581	158	0.10	0.10	0.5	13	1121
0	Tr	0.1	2	Tr	13	1	26	3	Tr	Tr	Tr	Tr	1122
0	11	7.5	102	2.7	852	49	1,779	178	0.25	0.16	1.0	21	1123
0	1	0.8	10	0.3	87	5	182	18	0.03	0.02	0.1	2	1124
0	Tr	0.2	7	0.1	26	1	190	19	0.01	0.01	Tr	2	1125
0	2	1.1	38	0.8	148	5	1,064	106	0.03	0.04	0.2	10	1126
0	Tr	0.2	4	0.1	29	1	260	26	0.01	0.01	0.1	2	1127
0	1	1.0	20	0.6	162	4	1,456	146	0.06	0.06	0.3	13	1128
0	3	0.8	4	0.7	259	3	0	0	0.06	0.30	2.8	2	1129
0	8	3.4	9	2.7	555	3	0	0	0.11	0.47	7.0	6	1130
0	8	3.7	17	1.2	201	663	0	0	0.13	0.03	2.5	0	1131
0	21	3.0	4	0.6	170	6	0	0	0.05	0.25	2.2	Tr	1132
0	3	0.4	Tr	0.1	55	Tr	0	0	0.01	0.05	0.5	Tr	1133
0	3	2.8	104	1.0	283	22	4,243	424	0.06	0.09	0.6	35	1134
0	12	4.0	101	0.7	515	8	920	93	0.21	0.09	1.4	26	1135
0	11	5.2	177	1.2	431	6	946	94	0.18	0.23	1.4	22	1136
0	14	2.9	32	0.4	251	5	0	0	0.07	0.03	0.2	10	1137
0	9	2.0	22	0.2	173	3	0	0	0.05	0.02	0.2	7	1138
0	1	0.3	3	Tr	22	Tr	0	0	0.01	Tr	Tr	1	1139

Table 9. Nutritive Value of the Edible Part of Food

Food No.	Food Description	Measure of edible portion	Weight (g)	Water (%)	Calories (kcal)	Protein (g)	Total fat (g)	Fatty acids Saturated (g)	Fatty acids Mono-unsaturated (g)	Fatty acids Poly-unsaturated (g)
	Vegetables and Vegetable Products (continued)									
1140	Cooked (whole or sliced), drained	1 cup	210	88	92	3	Tr	0.1	0.1	0.2
1141		1 medium	94	88	41	1	Tr	Tr	Tr	0.1
1142	Dehydrated flakes	1 tbsp	5	4	17	Tr	Tr	Tr	Tr	Tr
	Onions, spring, raw, top and bulb									
1143	Chopped	1 cup	100	90	32	2	Tr	Tr	Tr	0.1
1144	Whole, medium, 4⅛" long	1 whole	15	90	5	Tr	Tr	Tr	Tr	Tr
1145	Onion rings, 2"-3" dia, breaded, par fried, frozen, oven heated	10 rings	60	29	244	3	16	5.2	6.5	3.1
1146	Parsley, raw	10 sprigs	10	88	4	Tr	Tr	Tr	Tr	Tr
1147	Parsnips, sliced, cooked, drained	1 cup	156	78	126	2	Tr	0.1	0.2	0.1
	Peas, edible pod, cooked, drained									
1148	From raw	1 cup	160	89	67	5	Tr	0.1	Tr	0.2
1149	From frozen	1 cup	160	87	83	6	1	0.1	0.1	0.3
	Peas, green									
1150	Canned, drained	1 cup	170	82	117	8	1	0.1	0.1	0.3
1151	Frozen, boiled, drained	1 cup	160	80	125	8	Tr	0.1	Tr	0.2
	Peppers									
	Hot chili, raw									
1152	Green	1 pepper	45	88	18	1	Tr	Tr	Tr	Tr
1153	Red	1 pepper	45	88	18	1	Tr	Tr	Tr	Tr
1154	Jalapeno, canned, sliced, solids and liquids	¼ cup	26	89	7	Tr	Tr	Tr	Tr	0.1
	Sweet (2¾" long, 2½" dia)									
	Raw									
	Green									
1155	Chopped	1 cup	149	92	40	1	Tr	Tr	Tr	0.2
1156	Ring (¼" thick)	1 ring	10	92	3	Tr	Tr	Tr	Tr	Tr
1157	Whole (2¾" x 2½")	1 pepper	119	92	32	1	Tr	Tr	Tr	0.1
	Red									
1158	Chopped	1 cup	149	92	40	1	Tr	Tr	Tr	0.2
1159	Whole (2¾" x 2½")	1 pepper	119	92	32	1	Tr	Tr	Tr	0.1
	Cooked, drained, chopped									
1160	Green	1 cup	136	92	38	1	Tr	Tr	Tr	0.1
1161	Red	1 cup	136	92	38	1	Tr	Tr	Tr	0.1
1162	Pimento, canned	1 tbsp	12	93	3	Tr	Tr	Tr	Tr	Tr
	Potatoes									
	Baked (2⅓" x 4¾")									
1163	With skin	1 potato	202	71	220	5	Tr	0.1	Tr	0.1
1164	Flesh only	1 potato	156	75	145	3	Tr	Tr	Tr	0.1
1165	Skin only	1 skin	58	47	115	2	Tr	Tr	Tr	Tr
	Boiled (2½" dia)									
1166	Peeled after boiling	1 potato	136	77	118	3	Tr	Tr	Tr	0.1
1167	Peeled before boiling	1 potato	135	77	116	2	Tr	Tr	Tr	0.1
1168		1 cup	156	77	134	3	Tr	Tr	Tr	0.1
	Potato products, prepared									
	Au gratin									
1169	From dry mix, with whole milk, butter	1 cup	245	79	228	6	10	6.3	2.9	0.3
1170	From home recipe, with butter	1 cup	245	74	323	12	19	11.6	5.3	0.7
1171	French fried, frozen, oven heated	10 strips	50	57	100	2	4	0.6	2.4	0.4

Choles-terol (mg)	Carbo-hydrate (g)	Total dietary fiber (g)	Calcium (mg)	Iron (mg)	Potas-sium (mg)	Sodium (mg)	Vitamin A		Thiamin (mg)	Ribo-flavin (mg)	Niacin (mg)	Ascor-bic acid (mg)	Food No.
							(IU)	(RE)					
0	21	2.9	46	0.5	349	6	0	0	0.09	0.05	0.3	11	1140
0	10	1.3	21	0.2	156	3	0	0	0.04	0.02	0.2	5	1141
0	4	0.5	13	0.1	81	1	0	0	0.03	0.01	Tr	4	1142
0	7	2.6	72	1.5	276	16	385	39	0.06	0.08	0.5	19	1143
0	1	0.4	11	0.2	41	2	58	6	0.01	0.01	0.1	3	1144
0	23	0.8	19	1.0	77	225	135	14	0.17	0.08	2.2	1	1145
0	1	0.3	14	0.6	55	6	520	52	0.01	0.01	0.1	13	1146
0	30	6.2	58	0.9	573	16	0	0	0.13	0.08	1.1	20	1147
0	11	4.5	67	3.2	384	6	210	21	0.20	0.12	0.9	77	1148
0	14	5.0	94	3.8	347	8	267	27	0.10	0.19	0.9	35	1149
0	21	7.0	34	1.6	294	428	1,306	131	0.21	0.13	1.2	16	1150
0	23	8.8	38	2.5	269	139	1,069	107	0.45	0.16	2.4	16	1151
0	4	0.7	8	0.5	153	3	347	35	0.04	0.04	0.4	109	1152
0	4	0.7	8	0.5	153	3	4,838	484	0.04	0.04	0.4	109	1153
0	1	0.7	6	0.5	50	434	442	44	0.01	0.01	0.1	3	1154
0	10	2.7	13	0.7	264	3	942	94	0.10	0.04	0.8	133	1155
0	1	0.2	1	Tr	18	Tr	63	6	0.01	Tr	0.1	9	1156
0	8	2.1	11	0.5	211	2	752	75	0.08	0.04	0.6	106	1157
0	10	3.0	13	0.7	264	3	8,493	849	0.10	0.04	0.8	283	1158
0	8	2.4	11	0.5	211	2	6,783	678	0.08	0.04	0.6	226	1159
0	9	1.6	12	0.6	226	3	805	80	0.08	0.04	0.6	101	1160
0	9	1.6	12	0.6	226	3	5,114	511	0.08	0.04	0.6	233	1161
0	1	0.2	1	0.2	19	2	319	32	Tr	0.01	0.1	10	1162
0	51	4.8	20	2.7	844	16	0	0	0.22	0.07	3.3	26	1163
0	34	2.3	8	0.5	610	8	0	0	0.16	0.03	2.2	20	1164
0	27	4.6	20	4.1	332	12	0	0	0.07	0.06	1.8	8	1165
0	27	2.4	7	0.4	515	5	0	0	0.14	0.03	2.0	18	1166
0	27	2.4	11	0.4	443	7	0	0	0.13	0.03	1.8	10	1167
0	31	2.8	12	0.5	512	8	0	0	0.15	0.03	2.0	12	2268
37	31	2.2	203	0.8	537	1,076	522	76	0.05	0.20	2.3	8	1169
56	28	4.4	292	1.6	970	1,061	647	93	0.16	0.28	2.4	24	1170
0	16	1.6	4	0.6	209	15	0	0	0.06	0.01	1.0	5	1171

Table 9. Nutritive Value of the Edible Part of Food

Food No.	Food Description	Measure of edible portion	Weight (g)	Water (%)	Calories (kcal)	Protein (g)	Total fat (g)	Fatty acids Saturated (g)	Fatty acids Mono-unsaturated (g)	Fatty acids Poly-unsaturated (g)
	Vegetables and Vegetable Products (continued)									
	Potato products, prepared (continued)									
	Hashed brown									
1172	From frozen (about 3" x 1½" x ½")	1 patty	29	56	63	1	3	1.3	1.5	0.4
1173	From home recipe	1 cup	156	62	326	4	22	8.5	9.7	2.5
	Mashed									
1174	From dehydrated flakes (without milk); whole milk, butter, and salt added	1 cup	210	76	237	4	12	7.2	3.3	0.5
	From home recipe									
1175	With whole milk	1 cup	210	78	162	4	1	0.7	0.3	0.1
1176	With whole milk and margarine	1 cup	210	76	223	4	9	2.2	3.7	2.5
1177	Potato pancakes, home prepared	1 pancake	76	47	207	5	12	2.3	3.5	5.0
1178	Potato puffs, from frozen	10 puffs	79	53	175	3	8	4.0	3.4	0.6
1179	Potato salad, home prepared	1 cup	250	76	358	7	21	3.6	6.2	9.3
	Scalloped									
1180	From dry mix, with whole milk, butter	1 cup	245	79	228	5	11	6.5	3.0	0.5
1181	From home recipe, with butter	1 cup	245	81	211	7	9	5.5	2.5	0.4
	Pumpkin									
1182	Cooked, mashed	1 cup	245	94	49	2	Tr	0.1	Tr	Tr
1183	Canned	1 cup	245	90	83	3	1	0.4	0.1	Tr
1184	Radishes, raw (¾" to 1" dia)	1 radish	5	95	1	Tr	Tr	Tr	Tr	Tr
1185	Rutabagas, cooked, drained, cubes	1 cup	170	89	66	2	Tr	Tr	Tr	0.2
1186	Sauerkraut, canned, solids and liquid	1 cup	236	93	45	2	Tr	0.1	Tr	0.1
	Seaweed									
1187	Kelp, raw	2 tbsp	10	82	4	Tr	Tr	Tr	Tr	Tr
1188	Spirulina, dried	1 tbsp	1	5	3	1	Tr	Tr	Tr	Tr
1189	Shallots, raw, chopped	1 tbsp	10	80	7	Tr	Tr	Tr	Tr	Tr
1190	Soybeans, green, cooked, drained	1 cup	180	69	254	22	12	1.3	2.2	5.4
	Spinach									
	Raw									
1191	Chopped	1 cup	30	92	7	1	Tr	Tr	Tr	Tr
1192	Leaf	1 leaf	10	92	2	Tr	Tr	Tr	Tr	Tr
	Cooked, drained									
1193	From raw	1 cup	180	91	41	5	Tr	0.1	Tr	0.2
1194	From frozen (chopped or leaf)	1 cup	190	90	53	6	Tr	0.1	Tr	0.2
1195	Canned, drained	1 cup	214	92	49	6	1	0.2	Tr	0.4
	Squash									
	Summer (all varieties), sliced									
1196	Raw	1 cup	113	94	23	1	Tr	Tr	Tr	0.1
1197	Cooked, drained	1 cup	180	94	36	2	1	0.1	Tr	0.2
1198	Winter (all varieties), baked, cubes	1 cup	205	89	80	2	1	0.3	0.1	0.5
1199	Winter, butternut, frozen, cooked, mashed	1 cup	240	88	94	3	Tr	Tr	Tr	0.1
	Sweetpotatoes									
	Cooked (2" dia, 5" long raw)									
1200	Baked, with skin	1 potato	146	73	150	3	Tr	Tr	Tr	0.1
1201	Boiled, without skin	1 potato	156	73	164	3	Tr	0.1	Tr	0.2

Choles-terol (mg)	Carbo-hydrate (g)	Total dietary fiber (g)	Calcium (mg)	Iron (mg)	Potas-sium (mg)	Sodium (mg)	Vitamin A		Thiamin (mg)	Ribo-flavin (mg)	Niacin (mg)	Ascor-bic acid (mg)	Food No.
							(IU)	(RE)					
0	8	0.6	4	0.4	126	10	0	0	0.03	0.01	0.7	2	1172
0	33	3.1	12	1.3	501	37	0	0	0.12	0.03	3.1	9	1173
29	32	4.8	103	0.5	489	697	378	44	0.23	0.11	1.4	20	1174
4	37	4.2	55	0.6	628	636	40	13	0.18	0.08	2.3	14	1175
4	35	4.2	55	0.5	607	620	355	42	0.18	0.08	2.3	13	1176
73	22	1.5	18	1.2	597	386	109	11	0.10	0.13	1.6	17	1177
0	24	2.5	24	1.2	300	589	13	2	0.15	0.06	1.7	5	1178
170	28	3.3	48	1.6	635	1,323	523	83	0.19	0.15	2.2	25	1179
27	31	2.7	88	0.9	497	835	363	51	0.05	0.14	2.5	8	1180
29	26	4.7	140	1.4	926	821	331	47	0.17	0.23	2.6	26	1181
0	12	2.7	37	1.4	564	2	2,651	265	0.08	0.19	1.0	12	1182
0	20	7.1	64	3.4	505	12	54,037	5,405	0.06	0.13	0.9	10	1183
0	Tr	0.1	1	Tr	10	1	Tr	Tr	Tr	Tr	Tr	1	1184
0	15	3.1	82	0.9	554	34	954	95	0.14	0.07	1.2	32	1185
0	10	5.9	71	3.5	401	1,560	42	5	0.05	0.05	0.3	35	1186
0	1	0.1	17	0.3	9	23	12	1	0.01	0.02	Tr	Tr	1187
0	Tr	Tr	1	0.3	14	10	6	1	0.02	0.04	0.1	Tr	1188
0	2	0.2	4	0.1	33	1	119	12	0.01	Tr	Tr	1	1189
0	20	7.6	261	4.5	970	25	281	29	0.47	0.28	2.3	31	1190
0	1	0.8	30	0.8	167	24	2,015	202	0.02	0.06	0.2	8	1191
0	Tr	0.3	10	0.3	56	8	672	67	0.01	0.02	0.1	3	1192
0	7	4.3	245	6.4	839	126	14,742	1,474	0.17	0.42	0.9	18	1193
0	10	5.7	277	2.9	566	163	14,790	1,478	0.11	0.32	0.8	23	1194
0	7	5.1	272	4.9	740	58	18,781	1,879	0.03	0.30	0.8	31	1195
0	5	2.1	23	0.5	220	2	221	23	0.07	0.04	0.6	17	1196
0	8	2.5	49	0.6	346	2	517	52	0.08	0.07	0.9	10	1197
0	18	5.7	29	0.7	896	2	7,292	730	0.17	0.05	1.4	20	1198
0	24	2.2	46	1.4	319	5	8,014	802	0.12	0.09	1.1	8	1199
0	35	4.4	41	0.7	508	15	31,860	3,186	0.11	0.19	0.9	36	1200
0	38	2.8	33	0.9	287	20	26,604	2,660	0.08	0.22	1.0	27	1201

Table 9. Nutritive Value of the Edible Part of Food

Food No.	Food Description	Measure of edible portion	Weight (g)	Water (%)	Calories (kcal)	Protein (g)	Total fat (g)	Fatty acids		
								Saturated (g)	Mono-unsaturated (g)	Poly-unsaturated (g)

Vegetables and Vegetable Products (continued)

Sweetpotatoes (continued)

| 1202 | Candied (2½" x 2" piece) | 1 piece | 105 | 67 | 144 | 1 | 3 | 1.4 | 0.7 | 0.2 |

Canned

1203	Syrup pack, drained	1 cup	196	72	212	3	1	0.1	Tr	0.3
1204	Vacuum pack, mashed	1 cup	255	76	232	4	1	0.1	Tr	0.2
1205	Tomatillos, raw	1 medium	34	92	11	Tr	Tr	Tr	0.1	0.1

Tomatoes

Raw, year round average

| 1206 | Chopped or sliced | 1 cup | 180 | 94 | 38 | 2 | 1 | 0.1 | 0.1 | 0.2 |
| 1207 | Slice, medium, ¼" thick | 1 slice | 20 | 94 | 4 | Tr | Tr | Tr | Tr | Tr |

Whole

1208	Cherry	1 cherry	17	94	4	Tr	Tr	Tr	Tr	Tr
1209	Medium, 2⅗" dia	1 tomato	123	94	26	1	Tr	0.1	0.1	0.2
1210	Canned, solids and liquid	1 cup	240	94	46	2	Tr	Tr	Tr	0.1

Sun dried

1211	Plain	1 piece	2	15	5	Tr	Tr	Tr	Tr	Tr
1212	Packed in oil, drained	1 piece	3	54	6	Tr	Tr	0.1	0.3	0.1
1213	Tomato juice, canned, with salt added	1 cup	243	94	41	2	Tr	Tr	Tr	0.1

Tomato products, canned

1214	Paste	1 cup	262	74	215	10	1	0.2	0.2	0.6
1215	Puree	1 cup	250	87	100	4	Tr	0.1	0.1	0.2
1216	Sauce	1 cup	245	89	74	3	Tr	0.1	0.1	0.2

Spaghetti/marinara/pasta sauce. See Soups, Sauces, and Gravies.

| 1217 | Stewed | 1 cup | 255 | 91 | 71 | 2 | Tr | Tr | 0.1 | 0.1 |
| 1218 | Turnips, cooked, cubes | 1 cup | 156 | 94 | 33 | 1 | Tr | Tr | Tr | 0.1 |

Turnip greens, cooked, drained

1219	From raw (leaves and stems)	1 cup	144	93	29	2	Tr	0.1	Tr	0.1
1220	From frozen (chopped)	1 cup	164	90	49	5	1	0.2	Tr	0.3
1221	Vegetable juice cocktail, canned	1 cup	242	94	46	2	Tr	Tr	Tr	0.1

Vegetables, mixed

1222	Canned, drained	1 cup	163	87	77	4	Tr	0.1	Tr	0.2
1223	Frozen, cooked, drained	1 cup	182	83	107	5	Tr	0.1	Tr	0.1
1224	Waterchestnuts, canned, slices, solids and liquids	1 cup	140	86	70	1	Tr	Tr	Tr	Tr

Miscellaneous Items

| 1225 | Bacon bits, meatless | 1 tbsp | 7 | 8 | 31 | 2 | 2 | 0.3 | 0.4 | 0.9 |

Baking powders for home use

Double acting

1226	Sodium aluminum sulfate	1 tsp	5	5	2	0	0	0.0	0.0	0.0
1227	Straight phosphate	1 tsp	5	4	2	Tr	0	0.0	0.0	0.0
1228	Low sodium	1 tsp	5	6	5	Tr	Tr	Tr	Tr	Tr
1229	Baking soda	1 tsp	5	Tr	0	0	0	0.0	0.0	0.0
1230	Beef jerky	1 large piece	20	23	81	7	5	2.1	2.2	0.2
1231	Catsup	1 cup	240	67	250	4	1	0.1	0.1	0.4
1232		1 tbsp	15	67	16	Tr	Tr	Tr	Tr	Tr
1233		1 packet	6	67	6	Tr	Tr	Tr	Tr	Tr
1234	Celery seed	1 tsp	2	6	8	Tr	1	Tr	0.3	0.1
1235	Chili powder	1 tsp	3	8	8	Tr	Tr	0.1	0.1	0.2

Chocolate, unsweetened, baking

| 1236 | Solid | 1 square | 28 | 1 | 148 | 3 | 16 | 9.2 | 5.2 | 0.5 |
| 1237 | Liquid | 1 oz | 28 | 1 | 134 | 3 | 14 | 7.2 | 2.6 | 3.0 |

*For product with no salt added: If salt added, consult the nutrition label for sodium value.

Choles-terol (mg)	Carbo-hydrate (g)	Total dietary fiber (g)	Calcium (mg)	Iron (mg)	Potas-sium (mg)	Sodium (mg)	Vitamin A (IU)	Vitamin A (RE)	Thiamin (mg)	Ribo-flavin (mg)	Niacin (mg)	Ascor-bic acid (mg)	Food No.
8	29	2.5	27	1.2	198	74	4,398	440	0.02	0.04	0.4	7	1202
0	50	5.9	33	1.9	378	76	14,028	1,403	0.05	0.07	0.7	21	1203
0	54	4.6	56	2.3	796	135	20,357	2,035	0.09	0.15	1.9	67	1204
0	2	0.6	2	0.2	91	Tr	39	4	0.01	0.01	0.6	4	1205
0	8	2.0	9	0.8	400	16	1,121	112	0.11	0.09	1.1	34	1206
0	1	0.2	1	0.1	44	2	125	12	0.01	0.01	0.1	4	1207
0	1	0.2	1	0.1	38	2	106	11	0.01	0.01	0.1	3	1208
0	6	1.4	6	0.6	273	11	766	76	0.07	0.06	0.8	23	1209
0	10	2.4	72	1.3	530	355	1,428	144	0.11	0.07	1.8	34	1210
0	1	0.2	2	0.2	69	42	17	2	0.01	0.01	0.2	1	1211
0	1	0.2	1	0.1	47	8	39	4	0.01	0.01	0.1	3	1212
0	10	1.0	22	1.4	535	877	1,351	136	0.11	0.08	1.6	44	1213
0	51	10.7	92	5.1	2,455	231	6,406	639	0.41	0.50	8.4	111	1214
0	24	5.0	43	3.1	1,065	85*	3,188	320	0.18	0.14	4.3	26	1215
0	18	3.4	34	1.9	909	1,482	2,399	240	0.16	0.14	2.8	32	1216
0	17	2.6	84	1.9	607	564	1,380	138	0.12	0.09	1.8	29	1217
0	8	3.1	34	0.3	211	78	0	0	0.04	0.04	0.5	18	1218
0	6	5.0	197	1.2	292	42	7,917	792	0.06	0.10	0.6	39	1219
0	8	5.6	249	3.2	367	25	13,079	1,309	0.09	0.12	0.8	36	1220
0	11	1.9	27	1.0	467	653	2,831	283	0.10	0.07	1.8	67	1221
0	15	4.9	44	1.7	474	243	18,985	1,899	0.07	0.08	0.9	8	1222
0	24	8.0	46	1.5	308	64	7,784	779	0.13	0.22	1.5	6	1223
0	17	3.5	6	1.2	165	11	6	0	0.02	0.03	0.5	2	1224
0	2	0.7	7	0.1	10	124	0	0	0.04	Tr	0.1	Tr	1225
0	1	Tr	270	0.5	1	488	0	0	0.00	0.00	0.0	0	1226
0	1	Tr	339	0.5	Tr	363	0	0	0.00	0.00	0.0	0	1227
0	2	0.1	217	0.4	505	5	0	0	0.00	0.00	0.0	0	1228
0	0	0.0	0	0.0	0	1,259	0	0	0.00	0.00	0.0	0	1229
10	2	0.4	4	1.1	118	438	0	0	0.03	0.03	0.3	0	1230
0	65	3.1	46	1.7	1,154	2,846	2,438	245	0.21	0.18	3.3	36	1231
0	4	0.2	3	0.1	72	178	152	15	0.01	0.01	0.2	2	1232
0	2	0.1	1	Tr	29	71	61	6	0.01	Tr	0.1	1	1233
0	1	0.2	35	0.9	28	3	1	Tr	0.01	0.01	0.1	Tr	1234
0	1	0.9	7	0.4	50	26	908	91	0.01	0.02	0.2	2	1235
0	8	4.4	21	1.8	236	4	28	3	0.02	0.05	0.3	0	1236
0	10	5.1	15	1.2	331	3	3	Tr	0.01	0.08	0.6	0	1237

Table 9. Nutritive Value of the Edible Part of Food

Food No.	Food Description	Measure of edible portion	Weight (g)	Water (%)	Calories (kcal)	Protein (g)	Total fat (g)	Fatty acids		
								Saturated (g)	Mono-unsaturated (g)	Poly-unsaturated (g)

Miscellaneous Items (continued)

Food No.	Food Description	Measure of edible portion	Weight (g)	Water (%)	Calories (kcal)	Protein (g)	Total fat (g)	Saturated (g)	Mono-unsaturated (g)	Poly-unsaturated (g)
1238	Cinnamon	1 tsp	2	10	6	Tr	Tr	Tr	Tr	Tr
1239	Cocoa powder, unsweetened	1 cup	86	3	197	17	12	6.9	3.9	0.4
1240		1 tbsp	5	3	12	1	1	0.4	0.2	Tr
1241	Cream of tartar	1 tsp	3	2	8	0	0	0.0	0.0	0.0
1242	Curry powder	1 tsp	2	10	7	Tr	Tr	Tr	0.1	0.1
1243	Garlic powder	1 tsp	3	6	9	Tr	Tr	Tr	Tr	Tr
1244	Horseradish, prepared	1 tsp	5	85	2	Tr	Tr	Tr	Tr	Tr
1245	Mustard, prepared, yellow	1 tsp or 1 packet	5	82	3	Tr	Tr	Tr	0.1	Tr
	Olives, canned									
1246	Pickled, green	5 medium	17	78	20	Tr	2	0.3	1.6	0.2
1247	Ripe, black	5 large	22	80	25	Tr	2	0.3	1.7	0.2
1248	Onion powder	1 tsp	2	5	7	Tr	Tr	Tr	Tr	Tr
1249	Oregano, ground	1 tsp	2	7	5	Tr	Tr	Tr	Tr	0.1
1250	Paprika	1 tsp	2	10	6	Tr	Tr	Tr	Tr	0.2
1251	Parsley, dried	1 tbsp	1	9	4	Tr	Tr	Tr	Tr	Tr
1252	Pepper, black	1 tsp	2	11	5	Tr	Tr	Tr	Tr	Tr
	Pickles, cucumber									
1253	Dill, whole, medium (3¾" long)	1 pickle	65	92	12	Tr	Tr	Tr	Tr	0.1
1254	Fresh (bread and butter pickles), slices 1½" dia, ¼" thick	3 slices	24	79	18	Tr	Tr	Tr	Tr	Tr
1255	Pickle relish, sweet	1 tbsp	15	62	20	Tr	Tr	Tr	Tr	Tr
1256	Pork skins/rinds, plain	1 oz	28	2	155	17	9	3.2	4.2	1.0
	Potato chips									
	Regular									
	Plain									
1257	Salted	1 oz	28	2	152	2	10	3.1	2.8	3.5
1258	Unsalted	1 oz	28	2	152	2	10	3.1	2.8	3.5
1259	Barbecue flavor	1 oz	28	2	139	2	9	2.3	1.9	4.6
1260	Sour cream and onion flavor	1 oz	28	2	151	2	10	2.5	1.7	4.9
1261	Reduced fat	1 oz	28	1	134	2	6	1.2	1.4	3.1
1262	Fat free, made with olestra	1 oz	28	2	75	2	Tr	Tr	0.1	0.1
	Made from dried potatoes									
1263	Plain	1 oz	28	1	158	2	11	2.7	2.1	5.7
1264	Sour cream and onion flavor	1 oz	28	2	155	2	10	2.7	2.0	5.3
1265	Reduced fat	1 oz	28	1	142	2	7	1.5	1.7	3.8
1266	Salt	1 tsp	6	Tr	0	0	0	0.0	0.0	0.0
	Trail mix									
1267	Regular, with raisins, chocolate chips, salted nuts and seeds	1 cup	146	7	707	21	47	8.9	19.8	16.5
1268	Tropical	1 cup	140	9	570	9	24	11.9	3.5	7.2
1269	Vanilla extract	1 tsp	4	53	12	Tr	Tr	Tr	Tr	Tr
	Vinegar									
1270	Cider	1 tbsp	15	94	2	0	0	0.0	0.0	0.0
1271	Distilled	1 tbsp	17	95	2	0	0	0.0	0.0	0.0
	Yeast, baker's									
1272	Dry, active	1 pkg	7	8	21	3	Tr	Tr	0.2	Tr
1273		1 tsp	4	8	12	2	Tr	Tr	0.1	Tr
1274	Compressed	1 cake	17	69	18	1	Tr	Tr	0.2	Tr

Choles-terol (mg)	Carbo-hydrate (g)	Total dietary fiber (g)	Calcium (mg)	Iron (mg)	Potas-sium (mg)	Sodium (mg)	Vitamin A (IU)	Vitamin A (RE)	Thiamin (mg)	Ribo-flavin (mg)	Niacin (mg)	Ascor-bic acid (mg)	Food No.
0	2	1.2	28	0.9	11	1	6	1	Tr	Tr	Tr	1	1238
0	47	28.6	110	11.9	1,311	18	17	2	0.07	0.21	1.9	0	1239
0	3	1.8	7	0.7	82	1	1	Tr	Tr	0.01	0.1	0	1240
0	2	Tr	Tr	0.1	495	2	0	0	0.00	0.00	0.0	0	1241
0	1	0.7	10	0.6	31	1	20	2	0.01	0.01	0.1	Tr	1242
0	2	0.3	2	0.1	31	1	0	0	0.01	Tr	Tr	1	1243
0	1	0.2	3	Tr	12	16	Tr	0	Tr	Tr	Tr	1	1244
0	Tr	0.2	4	0.1	8	56	7	1	Tr	Tr	Tr	Tr	1245
0	Tr	0.2	10	0.3	9	408	51	5	0.00	0.00	Tr	0	1246
0	1	0.7	19	0.7	2	192	89	9	Tr	0.00	Tr	Tr	1247
0	2	0.1	8	0.1	20	1	0	0	0.01	Tr	Tr	Tr	1248
0	1	0.6	24	0.7	25	Tr	104	10	0.01	Tr	0.1	1	1249
0	1	0.4	4	0.5	49	1	1,273	127	0.01	0.04	0.3	1	1250
0	1	0.4	19	1.3	49	6	303	30	Tr	0.02	0.1	2	1251
0	1	0.6	9	0.6	26	1	4	Tr	Tr	0.01	Tr	Tr	1252
0	3	0.8	6	0.3	75	833	214	21	0.01	0.02	Tr	1	1253
0	4	0.4	8	0.1	48	162	34	3	0.00	0.01	0.0	2	1254
0	5	0.2	Tr	0.1	4	122	23	2	0.00	Tr	Tr	Tr	1255
27	0	0.0	9	0.2	36	521	37	11	0.03	0.08	0.4	Tr	1256
0	15	1.3	7	0.5	361	168	0	0	0.05	0.06	1.1	9	1257
0	15	1.4	7	0.5	361	2	0	0	0.05	0.06	1.1	9	1258
0	15	1.2	14	0.5	357	213	62	6	0.06	0.06	1.3	10	1259
2	15	1.5	20	0.5	377	177	48	6	0.05	0.06	1.1	11	1260
0	19	1.7	6	0.4	494	139	0	0	0.06	0.08	2.0	7	1261
0	17	1.1	10	0.4	366	185	1,469	441	0.10	0.02	1.3	8	1262
0	14	1.0	7	0.4	286	186	0	0	0.06	0.03	0.9	2	1263
1	15	0.3	18	0.4	141	204	214	28	0.05	0.03	0.7	3	1264
0	18	1.0	10	0.4	285	121	0	0	0.05	0.02	1.2	3	1265
0	0	0.0	1	Tr	Tr	2,325	0	0	0.00	0.00	0.0	0	1266
6	66	8.8	159	4.9	946	177	64	7	0.60	0.33	6.4	2	1267
0	92	10.6	80	3.7	993	14	69	7	0.63	0.16	2.1	11	1268
0	1	0.0	Tr	Tr	6	Tr	0	0	Tr	Tr	Tr	0	1269
0	1	0.0	1	0.1	15	Tr	0	0	0.00	0.00	0.0	0	1270
0	1	0.0	0	0.0	2	Tr	0	0	0.00	0.00	0.0	0	1271
0	3	1.5	4	1.2	140	4	Tr	0	0.17	0.38	2.8	Tr	1272
0	2	0.8	3	0.7	80	2	Tr	0	0.09	0.22	1.6	Tr	1273
0	3	1.4	3	0.6	102	5	0	0	0.32	0.19	2.1	Tr	1274

Index for Table 9

A
Alcoholic beverages 14
Alfalfa sprouts 76
Almonds 52
Apple butter. See Fruit butter, apple.
Apple juice 28
Apples 28
Applesauce 28
Apricot nectar 28
Apricots 28
Artichokes 76
Asian pear 28
Asparagus 76
Avocados 30

B
Bacon 58
Bacon bits 86
Bagels 36
Baked beans 52
Baking powders 86
Baking soda 86
Bamboo shoots 76
Banana bread 36
Bananas 30
Barbecue sauce 70
Barley, pearled 36
Bean sprouts, mung 76
Bean with pork soup 68
Beans
    Dry 52
    Lima
        Immature 76
        Mature, dry 52
    Snap 76
Beef 56
Beef bouillon 70
Beef broth 68
Beef jerky 86
Beef macaroni 60
Beef noodle soup 68
Beef stew 60
Beef stock 70
Beer 14
Beet greens 76
Beets 76
Berries. See type.
Beverages 14-16
Biscuits 36
Biscuit with egg and sausage 62
Black-eyed peas
    Immature 76
    Mature, dry 54
Blackberries 30
Blue cheese 16
Blue cheese dressing 24
Blueberries 30
Bok choy. See Pak-choi cabbage.
Bologna 58
Bouillon 68
Braunschweiger 58
Brazil nuts 54
Bread 36-38
Bread crumbs 38
Bread stuffing 38
Breakfast bar 38
Breakfast cereals
    Hot type, cooked 38
    Ready to eat 38-42
Broccoli 76
Brown and serve sausages 58
Brownies 42
Brussels sprouts 78
Buckwheat flour 42
Buckwheat groats 42
Bulgur 42
Burrito 62
Butter 22
Buttermilk 20

C
Cabbage 78
Caesar dressing 24
Cakes 42-44
Camembert 16
Candy 70-72
Cantaloupe 32
Carbonated beverages 14
Carambola 30
Caramel candy 70
Carob 70
Carob flour 54
Carrot juice 78
Carrots 78
Cashew nuts 54
Catfish 26
Catsup 86
Cauliflower 78
Celery 78
Celery seed 86
Cereals, breakfast 38-42
Challah. See Egg bread.
Cheddar cheese 16
Cheese 16-18
Cheese sauce 70
Cheeseburger 62
Cheesecake 44
Cheese-flavor puffs or twists 44
Cherries 30
Chestnuts 54
CHEX mix 44

Chicken	66
Chicken potpie	60
Chicken soup	
Broth	68
Cream of	68
Stock	70
With noodles	68, 70
With rice	68
With rice and vegetables	68
Chickpeas	54
Chili con carne	60
Chili powder	86
Chili sauce. See Tomato, chili sauce.	
Chimichanga	62
Chips	
Corn	46
Potato	88
Tortilla	52
Chives, raw	78
Chocolate	
Baking	86
Candy	70-72
Chocolate-flavored beverages	14
Chocolate-flavored syrup or topping	74
Chocolate milk	70
Chocolate pudding	74
Cilantro, raw	78
Cinnamon	88
Clam chowder	
Manhattan	68
New England	68
Clams	26
Club soda	14
Cocoa	14
Cocoa powder, unsweetened	88
Coconut	54
Cod	26
Coffee	14
Cola-type beverages	14
Coleslaw	62, 78
Collards	78
Cookies	44-46
Corn chips	46
Corndog	64
Corn (hominy) grits	38
Corn, sweet	78
Corn syrup	74
Corned beef	56
Cornbread	46
Cornmeal	46
Cornstarch	46
Cottage cheese	18
Couscous	46
Cowpeas. See Black-eyed peas.	
Crab	26
Crab cake	26
Crabmeat	26
Cracked wheat bread	36
Crackers	46
Cranberries, dried, sweetened	30
Cranberry juice cocktail	16
Cranberry sauce	30
Cream	
Half-and-half	18
Light, coffee, or table	18
Sour	20
Whipped topping	18
Whipping	18
Cream cheese	18
Cream of chicken soup	68
Cream of mushroom soup	68
Cream of tartar	88
Cream products, imitation	20
Croissant	46
Croissant with egg, cheese, bacon	62
Cucumbers	80
Cupcakes. See under Cakes.	
Curry powder	88

D

Dandelion greens	80
Danish pastry	46, 62
Daiquiri	14
Dates	30
Diet carbonated beverage	14
Dill weed, raw	80
Doughnuts	46
Duck	66

E

Eclair	46
Egg bread	36
Egg substitute	22
Eggnog	22
Eggplant	80
Eggs	22
Enchilada	62
Endive, curly	80
English muffin	46
English muffin, egg, cheese, and bacon	62
Espresso coffee	14

F

Fast foods	60-64
Feta cheese	18
Figs	30
Filberts. See Hazelnuts.	
Fish. See also under type of fish.	
Fillet, battered or breaded	26
Sandwich	62
Sticks	26
Stock	70
Flounder	26

Frankfurter. See also Hot dog (fast food).
 Chicken 66
 Meat 60
French bread 36
French dressing 24, 26
French toast 48
Frosting 72
Frozen desserts
 Dairy 20
 Nondairy 72
Frozen yogurt 20
Fruit and juice bar 72
Fruit butter, apple 72
Fruit cocktail 30
Fruit drinks 76
Fruit-flavored soda beverages 14
Fruit juices 28-36
Fruit punch drink 16
Fruitcake 42
Fudge 72

G

Garlic, raw 80
Garlic powder 88
Gelatin dessert 72
Gin 14
Ginger ale 14
Gingerbread 42
Granola bar 48
Grape drink 16
Grape juice 32
Grape soda 14
Grapefruit 30
Grapefruit juice 30
Grapes 30
Gravies 70
Greens. See under type of vegetable.
Grits. See Corn (hominy) grits.
Ground beef 56
Ground turkey 66
Gumdrops 72
Gummy candies 72

H

Haddock 26
Halibut 26
Ham 58
Hamburger
 Ground beef 56
 Sandwich 64
Hard candy 72
Hazelnuts 54
Hearts of palm 80
Herring, pickled 26
Hoisin sauce 70
Hominy grits. See Corn (hominy) grits.

Honey 74
Honeydew melon 32
Horseradish, prepared 88
Hot dog (fast food) See also Frankfurter. 64
Hummus 54
Hush puppies 64

I

Ice cream 20
Ice cream sundae 62
Ice milk. See also Ice cream, light. 62
Ice pop 72
Icing. See Frosting.
Indian fry (navajo) bread 36
Italian bread 36
Italian dressing 24
Italian ices 72

J

Jams 74
Jellies 74
Jelly beans 72
Jerusalem artichoke 80

K

Kale 80
Kasha. See Buckwheat groats.
Kelp 84
Ketchup. See Catsup.
Kiwifruit 32
Kohlrabi 80

L

Lamb 56-58
Lard 22
Leeks 80
Lemon juice 32
Lemon-lime soda 14
Lemonade 16
Lemons 32
Lentils 54
Lettuce 80
Lima beans
 Immature 76
 Mature, dry 52
Lime juice 32
Liqueur, coffee 14
Liver
 Beef 56
 Chicken 66
Lobster 26
Luncheon meat 58-60

M

Macadamia nuts 54
Macaroni 48

Macaroni and cheese	60
Malted milk beverages	16
Mandarin oranges. See Tangerines.	
Mangos	32
Maple syrup	74
Margarine	22-24
Margarine-butter blend	24
Marinara sauce	70
Marshmallows	72
Matzo	48
Mayonnaise	24
Meatless burger	60
Melons	32
Milk	20
Milk beverages	20-22
Milk chocolate candy	70
Milk shake	22
Minestrone soup	68
Miso	54
Mixed fruit, frozen	32
Mixed grain bread	36
Mixed nuts	54
Molasses	74
Mozzarella cheese	18
Muenster cheese	18
Muffins	48
Mushroom soup, cream of	68
Mushrooms	80
Mustard, prepared	88
Mustard greens	80

N

Nacho cheese sauce	70
Nachos	64
Nectarines	32
Neufchatel	18
Noodles, chow mein	48
Noodles, egg	48
Noodle soup	68, 70
NUTRI-GRAIN cereal bar	48

O

Oat bran	48
Oatmeal bread	36
Oatmeal cereal	38
Ocean perch	26
Oils, salad or cooking	24
Okra	80
Olives	88
Onion powder	88
Onion rings	82
Onion soup	70
Onions	80
Orange juice	32
Orange soda	14
Oranges	32
Oregano	88

Oriental snack mix	48
Oysters	26

P

Pak-choi cabbage	78
Pancake syrup. See Syrup, table blend.	
Pancakes	48
Papayas	32
Paprika	88
Parmesan cheese	18
Parsley	
Dried	88
Raw	82
Parsnips	82
Pasta sauce	70
Pasta with meatballs	60
Pasteurized process cheese	18
Pasteurized process cheese food	18
Pasteurized process cheese spread	18
Peaches	34
Peanut butter	54
Peanuts	54
Pears	34
Pea soup	68
Peas	
Edible pod	82
Green	82
Split, dry	54
Pecans	54
Pepper or hot sauce	70
Pepper, black	88
Pepper-type soda	14
Peppers	82
Perch, Ocean	26
Pe-tsai cabbage	78
Pickle relish	88
Pickles	88
Pie crust	48
Pie filling	
Apple	28
Cherry	30
Pies, baked	50
Pies, fried	50, 62
Pimento	82
Pina colada	14
Pineapple	34
Pineapple-grapefruit juice drink	16
Pineapple juice	34
Pineapple-orange juice drink	16
Pine nuts	54
Pistachio nuts	54
Pita bread	36
Pizza	64
Plantain	34
Plums	34
Pollock	26
Popcorn	50

Popcorn cakes	50
Popsicle. See Ice pop.	
Pork	
Cured (ham)	58
Fresh	58
Pork sausage	60
Pork skins	88
Potato chips	88
Potatoes	82
Potato products	
Au gratin	82
French fried	82
Hashed brown	84
Mashed	84
Potato pancakes	84
Potato puffs	84
Potato salad	84
Scalloped	84
Pretzels	50
Provolone cheese	18
Preserves. See Jams and preserves.	
Prune juice	34
Prunes	34
Puddings	74
Pumpernickel bread	38
Pumpkin	84
Pumpkin seed kernels	54

R

Radishes	84
Raisin bread	38
Raisins	34
Raspberries	34
Refried beans	54
Relish, pickle	88
Rhubarb	34
Rice	50
Rice beverage (RICE DREAM)	16
Rice cakes	50
RICE KRISPIES Treat Squares	50
Rice pudding	74
Ricotta cheese	18
Roast beef	56
Roast beef sandwich	64
Rockfish	26
Rolls	50
Root beer	14
Roughy, orange	28
Rum	14
Russian dressing	24
Rutabagas	84
Rye bread	38

S

Salad, tossed (fast food)	64
Salad dressings	24-26
Salami	60
Salmon	28
Salsa	70
Salt	88
Sandwich spread (pork, beef)	60
Sandwiches. See under type of filling or Submarine.	
Sardines	28
Sauces	70
Sauerkraut	84
Sausages	58-60
Scallops	28
Seaweed	84
Seeds, edible. See under type of seed.	
Sesame seeds	54
Shakes (fast food)	64
Shallots	84
Sherbet	20
Shortening	26
Shrimp	28
Snap beans	76
Sodas. See Carbonated beverages.	
Sole. See Flounder or sole.	26
Soups	68-70
Sour cream	20
Sourdough bread. See French or vienna bread.	
Southern peas. See Black-eyed peas.	
Soy milk	54
Soy products	54-56
Soy sauce	70
Soybeans	54, 84
Spaghetti	50
Spaghetti bolognese	60
Spaghetti in tomato sauce with cheese	60
Spaghetti sauce	70
Spices. See type of spice.	
Spinach	84
Spinach souffle	60
Spirulina	84
Sprouts	
Alfalfa	76
Mung bean	76
Squash	84
Squash seed kernels	54
Starfruit. See Carambola.	
Steak	56
Strawberries	36
Stuffing. See Bread stuffing	
Submarine sandwich	64
Sugars	74
Sunchoke. See Jerusalem artichoke	
Sunflower seeds	56
Sweetpotatoes	84-86
Sweet rolls	50
Swiss cheese	18
Swordfish	28
Syrups	74

T

Taco, beef	64
Taco salad	64
Taco shell	52
Tahini	56
Tangerine juice	36
Tangerines	36
Tapioca, pearl, dry	52
Tapioca pudding	74
Tea	16
Teriyaki sauce	70
Thousand island dressing	24
Toaster pastries	52
Tofu	56
Tomatillos	86
Tomato	
Chili sauce	70
Juice	86
Paste	86
Puree	86
Sauce	86
Soup	68
Tomatoes	86
Tortellini	60
Tortilla chips	52
Tortillas	52
Tostada	64
Trail mix	88
Trout	28
Tuna	28
Tuna salad	28
Turkey	66-68
Turnip greens	86
Turnips	86

V

Vanilla extract	88
Vanilla pudding	74
Veal	60
Vegetable juice cocktail	86
Vegetable soup	68
Vegetables, mixed	86
Vienna bread	36
Vienna sausages	60
Vinegar	88
Vinegar and oil dressing	26
Vodka	14

W

Waffles	52
Walnuts, English	56
Water, tap	16
Waterchestnuts	86
Watermelon	36
Wheat bread	38
Wheat flours	52
Wheat germ, toasted	52
Whiskey	14
White bread	38
White sauce	70
Whole wheat bread	38
Wines	14
Worcestershire sauce	70

Y

Yeast, baker's	88
Yogurt	22

These 10 guidelines are intended for healthy adults and children 2 and older. Their purpose is to promote good health and reduce the risk of chronic diseases such as heart disease, cancer, diabetes, and stroke.

USDA Dietary Guidelines for Americans

AIM FOR FITNESS . . .

- Aim for a healthy weight.
- Be physically active each day.

BUILD A HEALTHY BASE . . .

- Let the Pyramid guide your food choices.
- Choose a variety of grains daily, especially whole grains.
- Choose a variety of fruits and vegetables daily.
- Keep food safe to eat.

CHOOSE SENSIBLY . . .

- Choose a diet that is low in saturated fat and cholesterol and moderate in total fat.
- Choose beverages and foods to moderate your intake of sugars.
- Choose and prepare foods with less salt.
- If you drink alcoholic beverages, do so in moderation.

Source: U.S. Department of Agriculture/U.S. Department of Health and Human Services

The Food Guide Pyramid can help you choose a variety of foods to help achieve a balanced diet. Selecting foods from each group will provide the many nutrients our bodies need.

Food Guide Pyramid
A Guide to Daily Food Choices

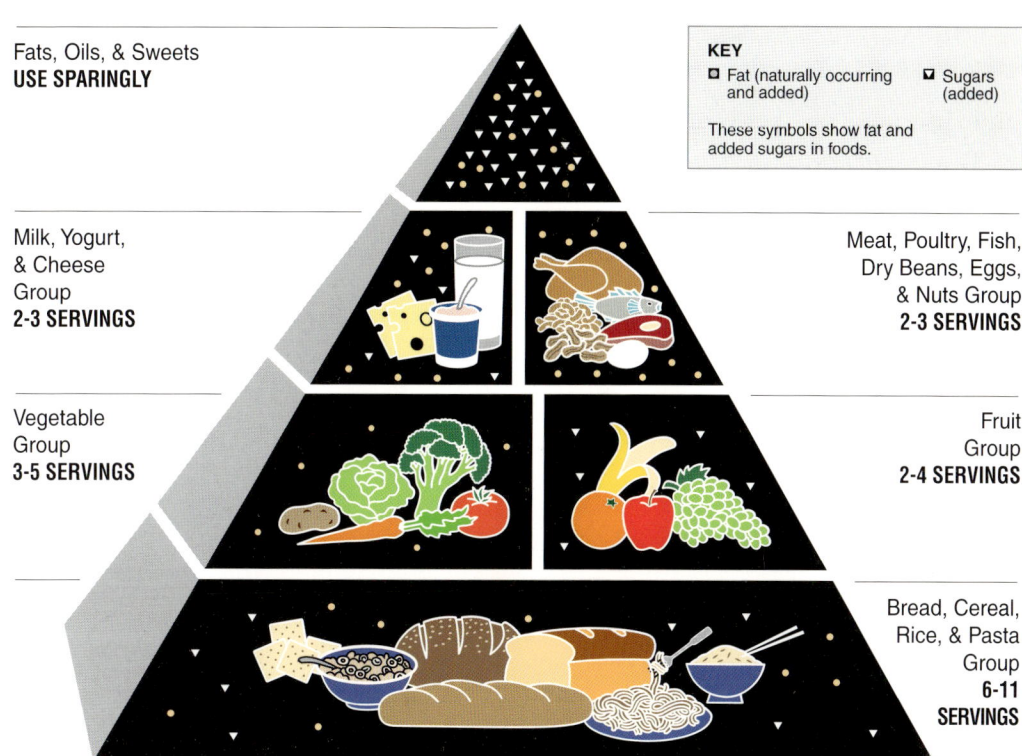

What Counts as One Serving?

The amount of food that counts as one serving is listed below. If you eat a larger portion, count it as more than 1 serving. For example, a dinner portion of spaghetti would count as 2 or 3 servings of pasta.

No specific serving size is given for the fats, oils, and sweets group because the message is USE SPARINGLY.

Milk, Yogurt, and Cheese
1 cup of milk or yogurt
1½ ounces of natural cheese
2 ounces of processed cheese

Meat, Poultry, Fish, Dry Beans, Eggs, and Nuts
2-3 ounces of cooked lean meat, poultry, or fish
1½ cup of cooked dry beans, 1 egg, or 2 tablespoons of peanut butter count as 1 ounce of lean meat

Vegetable
1 cup of raw leafy vegetables
½ cup of other vegetables, cooked, or chopped raw
¾ cup of vegetable juice

Fruit
1 medium apple, banana, orange
½ cup of chopped, cooked, or canned fruit
¾ cup of fruit juice

Bread, Cereal, Rice, and Pasta
1 slice of bread
1 ounce of ready-to-eat cereal
½ cup of cooked cereal, rice, or pasta

Source: U.S. Department of Agriculture/U.S. Department of Health and Human Services

ISBN 0-16-051197-6

90000

9 780160 511974